HIV and AIDS: A Very Short Introduction

VERY SHORT INTRODUCTIONS are for anyone wanting a stimulating and accessible way into a new subject. They are written by experts, and have been translated into more than 45 different languages.

The series began in 1995, and now covers a wide variety of topics in every discipline. The VSI library now contains over 500 volumes—a Very Short Introduction to everything from Psychology and Philosophy of Science to American History and Relativity—and continues to grow in every subject area.

Titles in the series include the following:

Alan Whiteside

HIV AND AIDS

A Very Short Introduction

SECOND EDITION

OXFORD
UNIVERSITY PRESS

OXFORD
UNIVERSITY PRESS

Great Clarendon Street, Oxford, OX2 6DP,
United Kingdom

Oxford University Press is a department of the University of Oxford.
It furthers the University's objective of excellence in research, scholarship,
and education by publishing worldwide. Oxford is a registered trade mark of
Oxford University Press in the UK and in certain other countries

First edition published in 2008
Second edition published in 2016

Impression: 3

Published in the United States of America by Oxford University Press
198 Madison Avenue, New York, NY 10016, United States of America

British Library Cataloguing in Publication Data
Data available

Library of Congress Control Number: 2016947261

ISBN 978-0-19-872749-1

Printed in Great Britain by
Ashford Colour Press Ltd, Gosport, Hampshire

Contents

Preface

It is over thirty years since clinicians in the United States identified the first cases of the syndrome that came to be known as AIDS. These initial reports simply referred to clusters of people with unusual illnesses. Today AIDS is a major killer of young adults globally. There are about 36.7 million people infected, the vast majority in developing countries. The number of people living with HIV continues to rise although new infections are declining.

I first took notice of HIV and AIDS in 1987 when researching labour migration in Southern Africa. Apartheid and the legacy of colonialism created the perfect hothouse for the spread of a sexually transmitted disease. What started as an academic and intellectual curiosity became intensely personal. The HIV prevalence in Swaziland, where I grew up, rose from 3.9 per cent among pregnant women in 1992 to over 40 per cent in 2004. I lived in South Africa where AIDS affected us all; we watched colleagues, friends, neighbours, and employees fall ill and die in the 1990s and early 2000s. We took these deaths in our stride. We welcomed the development of antiretroviral treatment that literally brought people back from the brink of death.

We have made huge progress in understanding the science of the virus: where it came from, how it works, how it spreads, and how it can be treated. In 2007, I wrote, 'we are still a long way from having a cure or vaccine', in 2016 this is closer, but not imminent. The main advances have been in treatment. We have the ability to prevent mother to child transmission (now called 'vertical transmission') and people can live near normal lives if they take the drugs. However, these remain relatively expensive, complex, and are not a cure. If patients do not adhere to treatment, the illness returns and their prospects are bleak.

This Very Short Introduction is about a unique and dynamic disease with long-term consequences. It provides an introduction to the science around the pandemic, focuses on the profound impacts AIDS had (and in some countries continues to have) on households, communities, and demographic and development indicators. It is very much clearer where AIDS will be a problem and why. The response has evolved but AIDS highlights deep philosophical questions about access to drugs and the value of life.

HIV and AIDS are a global phenomenon with the dynamics and consequences played out differently across the world. The burden is not borne equally. It is the deprived and powerless who are most likely to be infected and affected. AIDS is primarily a disease of the poor, be they nations or people. Geographically the worst epidemics are in sub-Saharan Africa, specifically Southern Africa, and many examples are drawn from here.

This VSI looks at the epidemic and what it means for countries, populations, production, and reproduction. AIDS calls on us to assess what is important to humankind, and how we relate to each other, both in our communities but also globally. It asks if it matters if a young Swazi girl has a greater than 50 per cent chance of dying from AIDS in her lifetime. What does it mean for older women caring for their children's children? The answers are not clear or simple. There are signs of hope; treatment is the good news. Nonetheless until the number of new infections falls below the number of HIV infected people dying globally and nationally—an AIDS transition—the epidemic will not end.

Writing the first edition proved more difficult than I would ever have believed. Preparing the second took longer than expected. It is being written when the end of AIDS may actually be in sight.

I would like to express my appreciation to many people for their help and support: the OUP staff in particular; in Durban the Health Economics and HIV/AIDS Research Division staff; in Canada my colleagues at the Balsillie School of International Affairs and specifically Nicholas Zebryk; my family Ailsa Marcham, Rowan Whiteside, and Douglas Whiteside; and many friends, colleagues, and readers, but specifically Professor Tony Barnett.

List of illustrations

List of tables

List of abbreviations

AIDS	Acquired Immunodeficiency Syndrome
ANC	antenatal clinic
ART	antiretroviral therapies
AZT	Azidothymidine
CBR	crude birth rates
CDC	Centers for Disease Control
CDR	crude death rates
CIHD	Centre for International Health and Development
DAH	Development Assistance for Health
DALYs	disability adjusted life years
DHHS	Department of Health and Human Services
DNA	deoxyribonucleic acid
DHS	demographic health survey
ELISA	Enzyme-Linked Immunosorbent Assay
GDP	gross domestic product
GF	Global Fund
GPA	Global Programme on AIDS
HDI	Human Development Index
HIV	Human Immunodeficiency Virus
IDU	intravenous drug user
MDG	Millennium Development Goal
MDR TB	multi-drug resistant tuberculosis
MTCT	mother-to-child transmission
NGO	non-governmental organisation
PEPFAR	Presidential Emergency Plan for AIDS Relief
RNA	ribonucleic acid
SARS	Severe Acute Respiratory Syndrome
SIDA	Syndrome d'immunodéficience acquise

SIV	Simian Immunodeficiency Virus
SSA	sub-Saharan Africa
STI	sexually transmitted infection
TAC	Treatment Action Campaign
TB	tuberculosis
TFR	total fertility rate
UNAIDS	Joint United Nations Programme on HIV/AIDS
UNDP	United Nations Development Programme
UNFPA	United Nations Fund for Population Activities
UNICEF	United Nations Children's Fund
USAID	United States Agency for International Development
WHO	World Health Organisation
XDR TB	extensively drug resistant tuberculosis

Chapter 1
The emergence and state of the HIV and AIDS epidemic

The identification of HIV and AIDS

Acquired Immunodeficiency Syndrome (AIDS) is caused by the Human Immunodeficiency Virus (HIV), which crossed from primates into humans. The first cases of the current epidemic probably occurred in the 1920s or earlier. Isolated transmissions may have happened before; but the disease did not get a foothold among humans. Rapid spread began in the 1970s.

AIDS was first publicly reported on 5 June 1981, in the Morbidity and Mortality Weekly Report (MMWR) produced by the Centers for Disease Control (CDC) in Atlanta in the United States. Doctors recorded unexpected clusters of previously extremely rare diseases such as *pneumocystis carinii*, a type of pneumonia, and Kaposi's sarcoma, normally a slow-growing tumour. These infections manifested in exceptionally serious forms, and, initially, within a narrowly defined risk group—young, homosexual men.

It soon became apparent these illnesses were occurring in other definable groups: haemophiliacs, blood transfusion recipients, and injecting drug users (IDUs). By 1982 cases were seen in the partners and infants of those infected. The name—'Acquired Immunodeficiency Syndrome'—was agreed in Washington in July

1982. AIDS describes the disease accurately: people acquire the condition; it results in a deficiency within the immune system; and is a syndrome not a single disease. The CDC produced a working definition for AIDS based on clinical signs. In French, Portuguese, and Spanish it is known as SIDA, the full French name being 'Syndrome d'immunodéficience acquise'.

Beyond North America there was news of cases from Europe, Australia, New Zealand, a number of African countries, Brazil, and Mexico. In Zambia a significant rise in cases of Kaposi's sarcoma was recorded. In Kinshasa, Zaire (now Democratic Republic of Congo), there was an upsurge in patients with *cryptococcosis*, an unusual fungal infection. The Ugandan Ministry of Health was receiving reports of increased and unexpected deaths among young people in Lake Victoria fishing villages.

Even when the syndrome had been identified and named, it was not immediately clear what its cause was, how it spread, and what treatments were effective or could be developed. Scientists agreed the most likely origin was an, as yet, unidentified virus. In laboratories across the world, the hunt to detect the cause was intense. In 1983 the virus was identified by the Institute Pasteur in France who called it '*Lymphadenopathy*-Associated Virus' or LAV. In April 1984 in the USA, the National Cancer Institute (NCI) isolated the virus and named it HTLV-III. There was an unfortunate spat when Margaret Heckler, the US Secretary of the Department of Health and Human Services (DHHS), announced to the world that the NCI was responsible for the scientific breakthrough that identified HIV. The face-saving compromise was to say French and US laboratories had both discovered the cause of the AIDS. In 1987 the name 'Human Immunodeficiency Virus' was confirmed by the International Committee on Taxonomy of Viruses. The current accepted terminology is HIV and AIDS, although where earlier work is quoted the term HIV/AIDS is retained.

Many diseases spread from animals to humans. These are called zoonoses. Recent examples include Severe Acute Respiratory Syndrome (SARS), tracked to civet cats; Avian Influenza (bird flu); Middle East Respiratory Syndrome (MERS), linked to camels; and the Ebola virus carried by fruit bats, which has been described as 'AIDS on steroids'. HIV is, so far, the most deadly pathogen to have made the leap across the species barrier to humans. SARS was, fortunately, not as infectious; avian flu has not yet taken hold in humans; MERS outbreaks have been infrequent and controlled. The Ebola outbreak is discussed later in the book.

Initially there was hysteria around AIDS, where it came from, and how it was transmitted. In San Francisco, when it was identified as a 'gay men's disease', police and fire officers feared they would be infected through exposure to blood and body fluids from homosexuals. They were given face masks and gloves and educated on protecting themselves from this assumed risk. Today when AIDS hits the headlines in the West, which is ever less frequently, most stories fall into a few categories: what the West (and Western celebrities) are doing to assist the worst affected countries and communities; the science of the epidemic; and, in rich countries, the deliberate spreading of the virus by individuals to implicitly 'innocent victims'.

Having identified how HIV was spread, the challenge was to reduce transmission. Early responses were technical: improving blood safety; providing condoms, and clean syringes and needles. Soon it became apparent these measures were not enough: behaviours needed to change. At the same time the race was on to find drugs to cure, or at least treat, infected people. It took fifteen years to develop effective antiretroviral therapies (ART). These were announced at the 1996 International AIDS Conference in Vancouver. There has been considerable progress with new and less toxic drugs being developed and the pill burden (the number of tablets an individual needs to swallow at specific times of the day in set combinations) being greatly reduced. However there is still not a cure.

There was little understanding of the potential long-term impact of the epidemic. While the worst predictions: of national collapse, rising crime, economic stagnation, and general malaise won't come about, vulnerabilities, like the epidemic itself, are differentiated. In some areas, nations are being adversely affected, in others the impact is limited to specific, usually marginalized, groups.

The long-wave epidemic

At the end of 2015, more than thirty years after the virus was identified, an estimated eighty-two million people have been infected with HIV, and of them over forty-one million have died from AIDS-related causes. The pattern of infections is discussed later. While no part of the world is untouched, modes of transmission and numbers infected vary greatly.

What makes HIV so distinctive is discussed further on. The virus itself is unusual; it comes from a retrovirus and is slow acting. The most common mode of transmission is sexual intercourse, followed by mother to child infection, sharing drug injecting equipment, and via contaminated blood or instruments in health care settings. Because transmission is mainly through sex or drug use and there is no cure, there was and is, prejudice and fear. HIV and AIDS remain stigmatizing at an individual and national level. This Very Short Introduction explores the consequences of increased illness and death, and the dramatic changes in treatment that have developed, and concludes by outlining the key issues and directions the disease may take us.

HIV and AIDS is a complex long-wave event. There are waves of spread and waves of impact. This concept is illustrated by the three curves in Figure 1. The first shows the prevalence rising

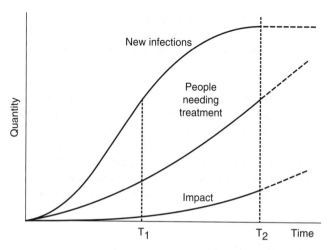

1. Epidemic curves.

steadily and levelling off, a silent spread. The second curve, six to ten years later, is the cumulative number of people requiring treatment. If treated they will not progress to death, but there are costs in keeping people alive and healthy. At T_1 the number of cases at T_2 needing ART can be predicted and planned for. The third curve, even further in the future, is the impact which is harder to forecast.

Some idea of the timescale comes from Uganda. Here HIV prevalence peaked in 1989–90 at about 14 per cent in adults. The number of AIDS orphans peaked in 2003–4. The diagram shows the three waves and over time it has become apparent there may be an oscillation. Uganda's prevalence fell to 6.4 per cent in 2006 then rose to 7.4 per cent in 2013. It is not clear if this rise will continue or be repeated in other settings: only time will tell.

The future of HIV/AIDS is, epidemiologically speaking, reasonably predictable. Unless the virus mutates and becomes more easily transmitted it will be contained. Science is advancing and new treatments are becoming available. Technological prevention methods—microbicides and vaccines—are in the pipeline, while medical male circumcision, proven to reduce transmission, is being rolled out in some settings.

The impacts are less certain but will be confined to the worst affected countries and most marginal groups. These countries are mostly African. Demographics of declining and ageing populations, and HIV infections in young adults, mean some Eastern European countries may be adversely impacted. However, in most countries, AIDS has evolved into just one of many challenges faced by governments, with infections found mainly in key populations.

The global and regional epidemics

Although most early reported cases were among gay men in the United States and Europe, the greatest numbers have consistently been African. In 1980 there were about 18,000 HIV infections in North America, 1,000 each in Europe and Latin America, and 41,000 in sub-Saharan Africa (although the true number was probably closer to one million).

There are different geographic sub-epidemics around the world. Table 1 shows current data. The global percentage of people aged 15 to 49 living with HIV rose from 0.3 per cent in 1990 to 0.8 per cent in 1999. It has remained at this level. In sub-Saharan Africa, 4.5 per cent of 15- to 49-year-olds are living with HIV; in Latin America and the Caribbean the figure is 0.5 per cent; in South Asia it is 0.3 per cent; while in the Middle East and North Africa it is 0.1 per cent.

There is variation within countries. South Africa had four population surveys carried out by the Human Sciences Research Council (HSRC), in 2002, 2005, 2008, and 2012. The entire population was sampled. The surveys found a national prevalence rate of 11.4 per cent in 2002; in 2005, 10.8 per cent; in 2008, 10.9 per cent; and 12.6 per cent in 2012. There was variation by province and place of residence. The highest prevalence in 2012 was in KwaZulu-Natal at 17.4 per cent, the lowest in the Western Cape at 5.1 per cent. In urban informal settings prevalence was 29.9 per cent and in urban formal areas 14.7 per cent.

There are 'key populations', people at greater risk. These include sex workers, men who have sex with men (MSM); and intravenous drug users (IDUs). The size of these populations and relative importance varies from country to county. Prevalence levels here are higher than in the general populations. In addition activities are often criminalized—especially sex work and drug use. Worryingly there are recent instances of homophobic legislation which further stigmatize MSM and HIV positive (HIV+) individuals.

Sub-Saharan Africa has the largest number of people living with HIV: nearly twenty-six million, just over 70 per cent of the global total. There are differences in the size and trajectory of African epidemics; but throughout the continent the main mode of transmission is heterosexual intercourse. Females account for 58 per cent of infections. In sub-Saharan Africa 'key populations' have higher prevalence. Median HIV prevalence in sex workers is 20 per cent compared with the global median of 3.9 per cent. Africa is home to the latest discriminatory actions against MSM. The twenty-two Global Plan priority countries established by the Joint United Nations Programme on HIV/AIDS (UNAIDS), are—except for India—all in sub-Saharan Africa. They are Angola, Botswana, Burundi, Cameroon, Chad, Côte d'Ivoire, Democratic Republic of the Congo, Ethiopia, Ghana, Kenya, Lesotho, Malawi, Mozambique, Namibia, Nigeria, South Africa, Swaziland, United Republic of Tanzania, Uganda, Zambia, and Zimbabwe.

The epidemic in sub-Saharan Africa can be divided into four distinct geographical areas. Southern African has the highest HIV

Table 1 Regional HIV and AIDS statistics, 2003, 2007, and 2014

Country	Adults (15+) and children living with HIV	Adults (15+) and children newly infected with HIV	Adults (15–49) prevalence (%)	Adults (15+) and child deaths due to AIDS
Sub-Saharan Africa				
2014	25.8 million	1.4 million	4.7	1.1 million
2007	22.5 million	1.7 million	5.0	1.6 million
2003	23.5 million	2.6 million	6.2	1.9 million
North Africa and Middle East				
2014	240,000	22,000	0.1	15,000
2007	380,000	35,000	0.3	25,000
2003	380,000	54,000	0.2	34,000
Asia				
2014	5 million	340,000	0.2	250,000
2007	4.8 million	432,000	0.3	302,000
2003	7.6 million	860,000	0.4	500,000
Latin America				
2014	1.7 million	87,000	0.4	47,000
2007	1.6 million	100,000	0.5	58,000
2003	1.4 million	130,000	0.5	51,000

Caribbean				
2014	280,000	13,000	1.1	11,000
2007	230,000	17,000	1.0	11,000
2003	310,000	34,000	1.5	28,000
Eastern Europe and Central Asia				
2014	1.5 million	140,000	0.6	53,000
2007	1.6 million	150,000	0.9	55,000
2003	1.1 million	160,000	0.6	28,000
North America, Western and Central Europe				
2014	2.4 million	85,000	0.3	27,000
2007	2.0 million	77,000	0.4	33,000
2003	1.8 million	65,000	0.5	30,000
TOTAL				
2014	36.9 million	2 million	0.8	1.5 million
2007	33.2 million	2.5 million	0.8	2.1 million
2003	36.2 million	3.9 million	1.0	2.6 million

Based on data taken from 'UNAIDS, Global Epidemic Report, 2006' and 'UNAIDS Factsheet 2015' <http://www.unaids.org/sites/default/files/media_asset/20150901_FactSheet_2015_en.pdf> with permission prevalence. In Botswana, in 2014, an estimated 25.2 per cent of 15- to 49-year-old adults were HIV+; in Lesotho the figure was 23.4 per cent; in South Africa, 18.9 per cent; and in Swaziland, 27.7 per cent. Malawi, Mozambique, Namibia, Zambia, and Zimbabwe have prevalences in the range of 10 per cent to 17 per cent. The East African countries of Kenya, Tanzania, Uganda, Rwanda, and Burundi have prevalences of 5.3 per cent, 5.3 per cent, 7.3 per cent, 2.8 per cent, and 1.1 per cent, respectively. In central Africa: Cameroon, both the Congos, and the Central Africa Republic are below 5 per cent while in West Africa and the Sahel it is below 3 per cent. Nigeria, with its 3.2 per cent prevalence, is slightly higher and is a concern because of the large population involved.

The main story for HIV and AIDS in the middle of the second decade of the 21st century is in Africa. The data from antenatal clinic (ANC) surveys in Figure 2 show prevalence reaching at unprecedented levels. Ironically as treatment improves and more people have access, death rates fall and prevalence rises.

The Caribbean has a limited number of countries with comparatively high prevalence: the Bahamas at 3.2 per cent, Belize at 1.5 per cent, Haiti at 2 per cent, and Jamaica at 1.8 per cent. In this region the bulk of new infections are through MSM: in Jamaica, 33 per cent of gay men are infected. In Latin America, 75 per cent of cases are in four countries: Brazil, Columbia, Mexico, and Venezuela; and 60 per cent of those infected are men. The key populations are MSM, female sex workers, IDUs, and transgendered women.

The Asian and Pacific epidemics are under control. Sex workers and their clients, MSM, transgendered people, and IDUs represent those who are most affected. Six countries: China, India, Indonesia, Myanmar, Thailand, and Vietnam account for more

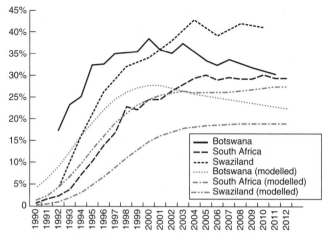

2. Actual HIV prevalence in antenatal clinics and modelled population prevalence.

than 90 per cent of the 4.8 million HIV infections. There is considerable variation in the 'most at risk' groups. In India overall, national prevalence among sex workers was estimated to be 2.8 per cent; in Mumbai specifically it was 22 per cent. Across the region the number of new infections has gone down everywhere except in Indonesia, where there has been a slight increase. A major concern continues to be IDUs. The epidemic can take off rapidly, but equally it can be quickly brought under control. In Cebu in the Philippines, HIV prevalence in IDUs rose from negligible levels in 2009 to more than 52 per cent in 2013. By contrast in Kathmandu, Nepal, among IDUs it fell from 68 per cent in 2002 to 6.3 per cent in 2011.

In the Middle East and North Africa reported prevalence levels are very low. The Islamic Republic of Iran and Sudan account for 30 per cent and 21 per cent of HIV infections, respectively. The main modes of transmission are IDUs, sex work, and MSM.

The number of new infections has increased, albeit only slightly in Sudan, Somalia, Morocco, Algeria, Egypt, and Tunisia.

In Eastern Europe and Central Asia there are an estimated 1.1 million people living with HIV, an increase of close to 200,000 since 2005. The epidemic here was driven by IDUs who in turn passed the virus to their sexual partners. The Russian Federation and Ukraine account for over 85 per cent of people living with HIV. Ukraine put in place extensive and effective prevention programmes involving needle and syringe programmes, and opioid substitution therapy. As a result the number of new infections among IDUs has fallen since 2008. Tellingly there are no data for Russia and other countries.

Western and Central Europe and North America have 2.3 million HIV infections, an increase of half a million since 2005, with 56 per cent in the United States. The burden of HIV is greatest among MSM, African American communities, and migrants from areas with high prevalence. African Americans make up 13.2 per cent of the population but account for 46 per cent of people living with HIV. The rate of new infections among heterosexual African American women is nearly double that of heterosexual men. The most at risk population are MSMs who represent 4 per cent of the male population but in 2010 accounted for 63 per cent of new infections.

In Europe the rate of new infections peaked in 2008. There were 29,157 new infections reported in in 2013. The greatest proportion were MSMs. Of the 32 per cent heterosexually transmitted, 11 per cent could be identified as originating in countries with a generalized epidemic. Just 5 per cent are from IDUs and the number of vertical transmissions was less than 1 per cent. The UK had the highest number of new cases at 5,993, followed by France with 4,002, Italy with 3,608, Spain with 3,278, and Germany with 3,263. (See Box 1.)

Box 1 Key features of the epidemic

HIV incidence and HIV prevalence have peaked. UNAIDS and the World Health Organisation (WHO) categorize four epidemiological scenarios:

- *Low-level*: here HIV has not spread to significant levels in any sub-population because networks of risk are diffuse. Rates of sexually transmitted infections and vulnerable and at risk populations should be monitored.

- *Concentrated*: prevalence is high enough in one or more sub-populations—such as MSM, IDUs, or sex workers and their clients—to maintain the epidemic there, but the virus is not circulating in the general population. The size of these vulnerable sub-populations and the frequency and nature of links between them and the general population determines spread.

- *Generalized*: where HIV prevalence is between 1 and 5 per cent in pregnant women attending antenatal clinics. The presence of HIV among the general population is sufficient for sexual networking to drive the epidemic. HIV transmission in sero-discordant couples and multiple partner relationships account for most new infections. Prevalence in most-at-risk populations will be higher. In an epidemic with more than 5 per cent adult prevalence, no sexually active person is 'low risk'.

- *Hyper-endemic*: HIV is above 15 per cent in adults in the general population, through extensive heterosexual, multiple concurrent partner relations with low and inconsistent condom use. All sexually active persons are at risk. The drivers include early sexual debut, long-term, multiple concurrent sexual partnerships—especially for men, inter-generational sex, gaps in condom use, low acceptability of condom use in couples, and biological co-factors such as low levels of male circumcision and the presence of sexually

Box 1 Continued

transmitted infections. There may be high levels of
HIV-related stigma, gender-based violence, including
sexual coercion and gender inequality.

As the epidemic has largely been brought under control there are
no instances of countries being 'promoted up' from categories,
although some have been 'relegated down'.

The maximum possible extent of the epidemic is clear. In 2002,
UNAIDS reporting on Southern Africa noted HIV prevalence had
reached levels 'considerably higher than previously thought
possible'. There is however a 'natural limit' beyond which
prevalence will not grow, when everyone who is likely to be
infected has been. The highest national prevalence recorded
among ANC attendees was Swaziland's 42.6 per cent in 2004. The
timing varies. Where the epidemic was reported early, in Uganda
and Thailand, by 1990 HIV prevalence had peaked and was
declining. In Southern Africa, HIV did not begin spreading
among the general population until the 1990s. In the former
Soviet Union the rapid increase began in the late 1990s.

The international dimension of the epidemic was not always
appreciated. Mobile populations provide an example of this.
Public Health England estimated in 2013 there were 107,800
people living with HIV in the UK. The Health Protection Agency
gave the source of infection. People of African birth accounted for
about 60 per cent of cases in 2003. Ten years later this proportion
had halved, however in 2013 black African men still accounted for
13,640 cases, 12.7 per cent of heterosexual cases; and black
African women for 25,060 heterosexual cases, 23.2 per cent of the
total. In 2013 Sweden 37.3 per cent of the admittedly small
number of 354 new HIV infections originated in sub-Saharan
Africa; in Norway the figure was 27 per cent; and in
Denmark, 17.6 per cent. Potential sources are migrant and

refugee flows, although nationals who travelled to source countries account for some cases. It is a complex and difficult problem, and reaffirms that HIV and AIDS are a global issue.

Prevalence and incidence

Prevalence and incidence are key concepts in epidemiology and important for this VSI. 'Prevalence' refers to the absolute number of people infected. The prevalence rate is the proportion of the population which has a disease at a particular time (or averaged over a period of time). With HIV, prevalence rates are given as a percentage of a specific segment of the population, for example adults aged between 15 and 49, ANC patients, blood donors, or the 'at risk' population. Data come from surveys—in the early years populations were blood donors, STD clinic patients, people with tuberculosis (TB), and pregnant women.

'Incidence' refers to the number of new infections over a given period of time. The incidence rate is the number per specified unit of population (this can be per 1,000, per 10,000—or million, for rare diseases) and time (in the case of cholera per day or week; for other diseases it could be per annum). Measuring HIV incidence was complex and expensive, but the new generation of tests can establish this, giving a better picture of the dynamics of the epidemic.

People infected with HIV remain so for the rest of their lives. The only way they leave the pool of HIV infections is by dying. This means the prevalence can continue rising even after the incidence has peaked. The introduction of ART makes understanding data more complex as, provided they adhere to treatment, people live longer. This is explored in Table 2. In this example incidence peaks in year six, and prevalence continues to rise. The introduction of ART in year nine means that prevalence rises more rapidly, but because treatment reduces viral load and thus the likelihood of transmission, the decline in incidence is faster.

Table 2 Incidence and prevalence

Year	Population	Incidence (actual)	Incidence rate per 1,000	Number of infected people (prevalence)	Prevalence rate (%)	Deaths of infected people	Comments
1	9,750	0		0			Year zero
2	10,000	50	5	50	0.5		
3	10,250	50	4.8	100	0.97		Slow increase
4	10,500	150	14.3	250	2.3		Exponential
5	10,750	550	51	750	6.9	200	
6	11,000	700	68	1,150	10.5	300	
7	11,250	650	57.7	1,400	12.4	400	
8	11,400	600	52.6	1,550	13.6	450	
9	11,400	400	35	1,750	15.4	200	ARVs introduced
10	11,300	300	26.5	1,850	16.4	200	
11	11,350	200	17.6	1,950	17.2	100	Prevalence rises
12	11,450	100	8.7	1,950	17.0	75	Prevalence stable

Where information comes from

The most consistent prevalence data came from women in ANC surveys, originally chosen because blood was routinely taken; the women had been sexually active; and the data could be anonymous and unlinked. The biases, intrinsic here, are that men were excluded; younger women over-represented as they are more likely to fall pregnant; HIV+ and older women under-represented as HIV infection and age reduce fertility; and surveys usually drew on women attending public clinics. This last point means women too poor to access the government clinics and those who get private health care are excluded. ANC data still give a reasonable picture provided biases are recognized.

Once data are available, it is possible to estimate the number and percentage of all women, men, and adults who are infected, as well as the number of babies at risk. This is done using models, some of which are in the public domain. Figure 2 shows actual and modelled data.

Increasingly the best data come from population-based surveys. These collect nationally representative HIV prevalence and provide information on characteristics associated with infection and risk. Most have been part of Demographic and Health Surveys (DHS). From 2001 to 2015 there were thirty-nine DHSs and six AIDS Indicator Surveys (AIS) carried out in African countries with generalized AIDS epidemics.

The surveys locate the epidemic by age and gender as the HSRC's data in Figure 3 shows for South Africa. Peak prevalence for women is in the 30 to 34 age group and for men it is those between 35 and 39. This gender and age distribution is typical of the heterosexual epidemics. A graph of most other countries would show more men than women infected as the epidemic is driven by IDUs and MSMs. The HSRC also provides data on race.

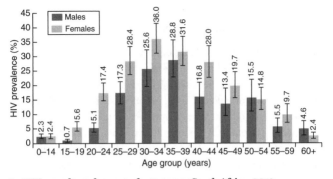

3. **HIV prevalence by sex and age group, South Africa, 2012.**

White prevalence in 2012 was 0.6 per cent; Indian or Asian origin, 1 per cent; mixed race, 4.6 per cent; and black, 22.7 per cent.

Growing sophistication of testing means additional data may be collected. This, in South Africa, included assessing for exposure to ART in infected individuals, a measure of how many people were on treatment. In the 2012 HSRC report, 2,002,000 of the 6,422,000 HIV infected people (31.2 per cent) were on therapy. Testing can measure incidence. In adults (15–49) incidence was estimated at 1.72 per cent, a slight decrease from the estimated 2.2 per cent in the 2002 to 2005 period. More significantly it fell from 5.3 per cent among females aged 15 to 24 in 2002–5 to 2.1 per cent in 2008–12. In Swaziland, the 2011 Swaziland HIV Incidence Measurement Survey (SHIMS) found incidence peaked among men aged 30 to 34 at 3.12 per cent; and among women aged 20 to 24 at 4.17 per cent.

The Institute of Health Metrics Evaluation (IHME) in Seattle produces data on burden of disease. It looks at disability adjusted life years (DALYs) lost from three broad categories of cause: communicable, newborn, nutritional, and maternal causes; non-communicable diseases; and injuries In 1990 HIV/AIDS ranked 33rd on the global list, by 2010 it was fifth. In sub-Saharan Africa it went from ninth to second over the same period.

It is believed global HIV incidence might have peaked, perhaps as early as the late 1990s. The number of new infections is falling. The issues are providing treatment; ensuring the trends are maintained; and reaching key populations.

Chapter 2
How HIV and AIDS work and scientific responses

AIDS appeared when the world was growing ever more interconnected, one of the main reasons it spread so rapidly. It also came at a time of unprecedented scientific advance and optimism. The eradication of smallpox in 1977, and advances in virology and immunology, and of other medical disciplines, raised expectations of what science and medicine could deliver. This chapter explains how HIV operates and is transmitted, and how science has progressed in the challenge to discover and deliver practical treatments and prevention measures.

Although the origins and mechanisms of HIV and AIDS were quickly understood, it became clear there was no medical or scientific silver bullet. Preventing HIV transmission and successfully treating patients needed more than laboratory work. The epidemic is lodged in parts of the world where poverty and inequity are rampant. The gendered nature of transmission and its location among marginal populations is critical. Dealing with this disease means understanding the science, and looking beyond it.

How the virus works

There are two main sub-types of the virus—HIV-1 and HIV-2—the latter being harder to transmit and slower acting.

Both originate in Simian (monkey) immunodeficiency viruses (SIV) found in Africa. The source of HIV-1 was chimpanzees in Central Africa while HIV-2 was derived in West Africa from sooty mangabey monkeys. How and when the virus crossed the species barrier continues to be a source of speculation and historical interest. Current thinking is the epidemic had its origins through chimpanzee and monkey blood entering peoples' bodies, probably during butchering of bush meat. The earliest plasma sample, subsequently found to have HIV, was taken in the Democratic Republic of the Congo in 1960. This led scientists to calculate the current HIV-1 epidemic originated in a zoonotic event in Cameroon between 1884 and 1924. HIV-2 crossed into humans in the 1940s.

Viruses have been described as 'a piece of nucleic acid surrounded by bad news'. A virus is genetic material covered with a coat of protein molecules. They do not have cell walls, are parasitic, and can only replicate by entering host cells. Viruses have few genes compared with other organisms: HIV has fewer than ten genes; the smallpox virus has between 200 and 400 genes; the smallest bacterium has 5,000 to 10,000 genes; and humans have about 30,000 genes.

The genetic material of life forms, including most viruses, is deoxyribonucleic acid (DNA). This contains the genetic instructions which specify the biological development of cellular life. Some viruses, including HIV, have ribonucleic acid (RNA) as their genetic material. They are called retroviruses (scientifically, retroviridae). HIV belongs in the family of viruses known as lentiviruses, that is, slow-acting.

HIV has to invade cells to reproduce. Within these it produces more virus particles by converting viral RNA into DNA before reproducing many destructive RNA copies. The conversion is done through an enzyme called reverse transcriptase. The switch from RNA to DNA and back to RNA is significant and makes combating HIV difficult. Each time it occurs there is a possibility of errors and the virus mutating or altering. This is made more likely because reverse transcriptase lacks the normal 'proofreading' that occurs with DNA replication. Once formed, the copies of virus particles break out of the cell, destroying it and going on to infect other cells.

The mutation of the virus enabled various sub-types or clades of virus to evolve. Identifying clusters or clades allows scientists and epidemiologists to track the spread of infection. Type B is the primary clade in the United States, type C dominates in Southern Africa, while in East Africa, types A and D are most common. The greatest variety is in West Central Africa.

Mutation equips the virus to outwit human responses and is one reason why a cure has not yet been found. This includes both our biological response and the technology we deploy through drug development. Individual human immune systems fight infections, and we can pass this resistance and response on to future generations. However, HIV undermines this ability by effectively targeting the cells of the immune system—and CD4 cells in particular.

There are two main types of CD4 cells. HIV primarily infects the CD4 T cells which organize the overall immune response to foreign bodies and infections. The virus also attacks macrophages, the immune cells which engulf foreign invaders in the body, and recognize, instruct, and equip the immune system for the future. Once the virus has penetrated the wall of the CD4 cell, it is safe as it masquerades as part of the immune system.

Some virus particles lie dormant in the cells until their replication is activated. The trigger could be an infection such as TB, or the deterioration of the immune system. The process of viral insertion, transcription, and particle expulsion is shown in Figure 4.

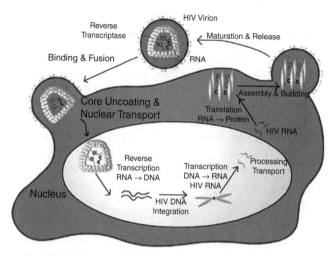

4. The HIV life cycle.

The virus mutates and becomes resistant to drugs. For an individual, this means the drug combination they take should be tailored to the variant of virus with which they are infected. This process is expensive and complex, requiring sophisticated laboratory facilities. At an individual level, a person developing drug-resistant HIV infection in the rich world can expect to receive costly tests and appropriate drug combinations; in the poor world, set combinations, known as first, second, and third lines of therapy are used. At the population level, drug-resistant infections have long-term ramifications; if they spread, treatment becomes much more difficult and expensive for everyone.

HIV mutation may mean the virus becomes less deadly. Equally, it could become yet more robust and easily transmitted. Virologists monitor the virus and its changes to ensure we are warned of new developments. While it is understood that HIV infection is incurable, what is not generally appreciated is that an HIV infected person can be re-infected with new strains of the virus, developing 'super infections'. (Box 2.)

Box 2 Testing

Most HIV tests look for the presence of antibodies not the virus: if a person has antibodies, they are infected. The most common test is the cheap and simple enzyme-linked immunosorbent assay (ELISA). Initially, HIV could only be detected using blood samples. The HSRC and DHS surveys described in Chapter 1 collected blood on absorbent paper by pricking a finger, heel, or ear. This is invasive, people don't like having blood taken, but it is as simple as the process diabetics go through to assess blood-sugar levels. Tests to identify antibodies in saliva (and other fluids) were developed, and are quick and easy to use.

Indirect tests such as the ELISA are cheap and quick. Testing for the virus is sometimes preferable, especially during early infection and in infants and children, when ELISA testing will not detect the virus. Direct testing involves a process called 'polymerase chain reaction' (PCR), using a technique by which DNA from a cell can be replicated until it can be measured. Both ELISAs and PCRs are used for detection of other diseases.

When a person is newly infected, they *sero-convert*—this means the virus has taken hold in the body. During this period, an infected person may experience a period of flu-like illness and will have a very high viral load: numerous virus particles in the blood stream or body fluids, especially semen or vaginal secretions. This is of epidemiological significance as immediately after infection, a person is hyper infectious. The more sexual activity or needle sharing by people in the early stages, the greater the chance of exposure and infection, thus the epidemic builds momentum. There is also a deceptive 'window period' when a person may be infected and infectious, and the virus not be detectable by ELISA tests. Thus, standard HIV tests are not completely reliable for new infections, blood supply safety cannot be absolutely guaranteed,

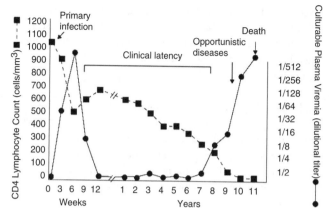

5. Viral load and CD4 cell counts over time.

and people wanting to be certain of their status should have two tests, three months apart.

The 'window period' is followed by the long incubation stage. During this phase, the viruses and the cells they attack are reproducing rapidly and are wiped out just as quickly by each other. Every day up to 5 per cent of the body's CD4 cells (about 2,000 million cells) may be destroyed by approximately ten billion new virus particles. Eventually, the virus destroys immune cells more quickly than they can be replaced. A healthy CD4 cell count is normally over 1,000 cells per mm^3 of blood. As infection progresses, this number falls, and the viral load increases, as shown in Figure 5.

Stages of infection

The WHO recognizes four disease stages based on clinical findings. First developed in 1990 and revised in 2007, these are intended to guide diagnosis, evaluation, and management of HIV and AIDS; do not require a CD4 cell count; and may be used in resource-constrained settings to determine eligibility for therapy.

Stages are categorized as 1 through 4. Stage 1 is asymptomatic infection. Stage 4, AIDS, occurs when the person is seriously ill with diseases such as extra-pulmonary TB, *Pneumocystis carinnii* and other pneumonias, the parasitic disease toxoplasmosis, and meningitis.

Viral load testing is increasingly available and less expensive, even in resource-poor settings. The WHO recognized the importance of viral load monitoring as early as 2003. Routine measurement is strongly recommended as the preferred way to diagnose treatment failure. These tests will become more available as costs fall, and technology is making them more robust and accessible.

Transmission

HIV is found in all body fluids of an infected person, although minimally in sweat, tears, and saliva. Exposure to blood or blood products carries heightened risk of infection. This is why there is so much concern for blood safety and hygiene in health care settings; and accounts for high levels of transmission among drug users who share syringes. Sexual intercourse is the most common source of transmission, accounting for over 75 per cent of all infections. Transmission occurs in both homosexual and heterosexual intercourse; globally, heterosexual transmission predominates. The second most important route of spread is contaminated drug injecting equipment, which is driving the epidemic in Eastern Europe and parts of Asia.

The virus can be passed from infected mothers to infants by crossing the placenta before birth, during delivery, and through breast milk. This is now referred to as 'vertical transmission' to avoid allocating blame to the mothers. Reducing the risk prior to or during birth is simple, even in most resource-poor settings, provided mothers are reached. The drugs are cheap and easily administered and lower the rate of transmission from the worst case scenario of 45 per cent to less than 5 per cent.

Table 3 Routes of exposure and risk of infection

Type of exposure	Risk per 10,000 exposures
Sexual transmission	
Receptive penile-vaginal intercourse (female risk)	8
Insertive penile-vaginal intercourse (male risk)	4
Insertive anal intercourse (male risk)	11
Receptive anal intercourse (male and female risk)	138
Fellatio	low
Parenteral transmission	
Blood transfusion	9,250
Needle sharing	63
Needle stick	23
Transmission from mother to infant	
Without treatment	1:4
With treatment	less than 1:10

'Estimated Per-Act Probability of Acquiring HIV from an Infected Source, by Exposure Act' from http://www.cdc.gov/hiv/policies/law/risk.html

The more complex question is what to do after the baby is delivered. The 2015 WHO guideline for pregnant and breastfeeding HIV+ women is that lifelong ART be provided regardless of CD4 count or WHO clinical stage. All HIV+ infants should receive ART. Identification of infected and uninfected infants is problematic, since early detection is difficult. The proposal is all infants born to HIV+ mothers in resource-poor settings should receive ART for three months and then be tested.

Those who are positive should continue treatment. These tests may need to be repeated. Women on treatment, who are ART adherent, have little chance of transmitting HIV through breast milk.

The comparative average efficiency of different modes of transmission is shown in Table 3. This shows that women are more at risk than men; and receptive anal intercourse is the riskiest behaviour regardless of the gender of the recipient. The chance of infection varies with stage of disease, and the viral load is crucial. Also important is the state of the immune system, health, and nutritional status of the exposed person. A major benefit of ART is it reduces the viral load, making a person on treatment much less infectious.

Treatment

In the absence of treatment, infections increase in frequency, severity, and duration until the person dies. The period from infection to illness is, on average, about eight years. This can be extended with basic lifestyle changes: eating a balanced diet; not smoking, not taking recreational drugs or excessive amounts of alcohol; and getting regular exercise. Immune system boosters, including some indigenous and herbal preparations, may help prevent opportunistic infections and prolong life. However there may be adverse interactions between these preparations and prescribed drugs once people start ART.

Nutrition, diet, and HIV are intimately linked. HIV can lead to malnutrition, while poor diet can in turn speed the infection's progress. A Malawian study found that patients with mild malnutrition were twice as likely to die in the first three months of treatment. For those with severe malnutrition the risk was six times greater.

An increasingly important question is how well the drugs work in people who lack food. People without sufficient nutrition may find that taking ART leads to unpleasant side effects and pain. Hungry individuals may skip treatment. The DHHS recommends that care for people living with HIV should involve a registered dietician with appropriate expertise. WHO advocates routine evaluation of patient's nutritional status and assessment of dietary intake.

Infected people have greater calorific needs. Asymptomatic adults and children require 10 per cent more energy from their diet than normal. Adults who have become ill need 20 per cent to 30 per cent more energy, while sick children require 50 per cent to 100 per cent more. Complicating factors for people suffering from AIDS are loss of appetite, inability to eat due to infections of the mouth and throat, and failure to properly digest food. If income falls due to illness there may be less food available in the household.

As the CD4 cell count falls and the immune system is compromised, the infected person experiences 'opportunistic' infections that rarely affect or cause serious symptoms in healthy people. Most infections can be treated, and the role of prophylaxis is important. An antibiotic such as cotrimoxazole prevents *Pneumocystis carinnii* infections. Other bacterial pneumonias, toxoplasmosis, salmonella bacteraemia, and TB can be prevented with isoniazid. These treatments are cheap and effective but don't address the underlying HIV infection.

Eventually ART is vital. These drugs reduce viral activity, allow the immune system to recover, and prolong and improve quality of life. In the USA in 1991 AIDS was the leading cause of death among adults aged 25 to 44, with rates reaching close to forty deaths per 100,000 by 1995. The introduction of ART in 1996 caused mortality to plummet. By 2000, it had fallen to about 10 per 100,000. Patients who had resigned themselves to death, cashing in life insurance policies and giving up employment, were granted a new lease of life so dramatic it became known as the 'Lazarus syndrome'.

The first effective drug was azidothymidine, known as AZT with the trade name Retrovir. This offered only short-term benefits as resistance to the drug developed rapidly. It was found that combinations of drugs, acting in different places and on different stages of the viral replication cycle (shown in Figure 4), were most effective, and standard treatment of triple therapy, using three different drugs, was developed. It does not eliminate the virus from a patient's body, and reservoirs of infection remain. If treatment ceases, the virus quickly remerges and begins replication.

The package of drugs offered in resource-poor settings, as a first line of treatment, includes two nucleoside reverse transcriptase inhibitors (NRTIs) plus a non-nucleoside reverse-transcriptase inhibitor (NNRTI) which stops HIV from replicating in cells. The WHO recommends that second-line therapy include two NRTIs with a third class of drug called protease inhibitors (PIs), which prevent viral replication. Third-line regimens include new drugs such as integrase inhibitors and second-generation NNRTIs and PIs, create minimal risk of cross-resistance with previously used regimens. Also available are drugs that prevent entry of HIV into the cells. In 2015 a potential new drug class—maturation inhibitors, which prevent development of immature HIV particles after they emerge from cells—was becoming available. The guidelines as to which drugs to use, and in which combination, will alter with scientific advances and changing prices.

There has been huge progress in drug development since ART was announced in 1996. Instead of taking handfuls of different tablets at specified times of the day it is possible for patients to take just one pill a day. The next major advance will probably be a weekly pill or injection and, eventually, an implant that lasts for months.

All the drugs used to treat HIV/AIDS are complex and relatively expensive (particularly PIs, some of which require refrigeration). They are also toxic. Not all patients can tolerate them, and not all drugs will work for an individual. Combinations and dosages are adapted accordingly. Few drugs are available in paediatric formulations.

There was a debate as to the best time to begin the ART regimen. The 2015 WHO guidelines are unequivocal: ART should be initiated in all HIV+ people no matter what their CD4 cell count is. Where there are not the resources to do this the WHO suggests prioritizing anyone in Stage 3 or 4 and those with a CD4 count ≤ 350. This is ideal, but there are issues of resources, equity, and returns. This is revisited in later chapters.

Western pharmaceutical companies are the main source of new drugs, while cheaper generic versions come from developing-world manufacturers, mainly in India. South Africa and Brazil are recent entrants into drug manufacturing. The major purchasers of drugs are agencies such as the US Presidential Emergency Plan for AIDS Relief (PEPFAR), the Global Fund for AIDS, TB and Malaria (GF), and national governments. Prices vary depending on who does the procurement.

Despite price reductions, affordability and access remain a life or death issue. In Uganda, combined public and private spending on all health care was only US$59 (current dollars) per capita in 2013; in Malawi it was US$26, and in South Africa US$593. In 2013, the average cost of first-line ART for low and middle income countries was $115 per patient per year (PPY); for second-line $330 PPY, and the price of third-line drugs was more than $1,500 PPY. These figures exclude clinical consultations, monitoring, tests, and drugs for opportunistic infections. If the state, aid agencies, NGOs, or faith-based organizations did not provide treatment, then it would be only accessible to the wealthy.

It is not only drug prices that create accessibility problems: poor people may not be able to afford transport to clinics, time off work, and the right nutrition. Poverty affects adherence to, and success of, treatment.

TB and HIV

The issue of TB and HIV is not fully understood outside medical circles. While most diseases that affect HIV+ people are not a threat to others, TB is a crucial exception. In 1990, AIDS was ranked thirteenth in the IHME's sub-Saharan African table of DALYs, TB was eighth. In 2013, AIDS was second while TB remained in the eighth spot. In 2013, nine million people developed TB and over 1.5 million died, 300,000 of these were HIV+. TB accounts for 25 per cent of all HIV-related deaths.

The WHO estimates that about one-third of the world's population harbours latent TB—people who have been exposed to the TB bacteria, but are not ill and do not infect others. On average, the lifetime risk of an infected person falling ill with TB is around 10 per cent. Conversely, HIV+ people are over one-quarter more likely to develop TB. Africa has the greatest proportion of new TB cases—280 per 100,000 in 2013. In North America between three and four people per 100,000 fall ill annually.

TB is generally treatable and curable with four antimicrobial drugs over a six-month period. However, without proper supervision and technical support, adherence to the treatment can be difficult and fail. There is also a growing concern about multidrug-resistant TB (MDR-TB), which is when bacteria do not respond to first-line drugs. Its development may be caused by ineffective treatment, incorrect use, or low-quality TB drugs and non-adherence. MDR-TB is more complex to treat, with lower cure rates and slower results—it takes two years, costs up to 100 times more, and it may be transmitted to others.

In 2006, there were reports from South Africa of an outbreak of extensively drug-resistant (XDR) TB, a form for which few drugs are effective. In Tugela Ferry hospital, of the 542 TB patients, fifty-three had XDR TB and fifty-two of these patients died within weeks of being identified; forty-four patients were tested for HIV and all were positive.

The WHO says that HIV and AIDS and TB are so closely connected that the terms 'co-epidemic' or 'dual epidemic' can be used to describe their interconnectedness. They have variously been referred to as 'the terrible twins' and 'Bonnie and Clyde'. Each disease speeds the progress of the other: TB shortens the survival time of people with HIV and AIDS. HIV+ people have increased likelihood of acquiring new TB infection, more rapid progression of latent TB, and relapses if previously treated. Having HIV makes the diagnosis and treatment of TB more complex and costly. Both diseases are more common in poor and marginal populations.

It is recommended that TB patients be offered voluntary counselling and testing for HIV, and that people who are HIV infected be tested for TB and treated or given prophylaxis. People who are on ART are less likely to develop TB. ART reduces the individual risk of TB and recurrence rate by over 50 per cent among HIV infected people.

The links between TB and HIV have the potential to make HIV a broader public health issue. Exposure to TB is more difficult to control since it is caused by airborne bacteria. In settings where large numbers of people are HIV+, a serious TB epidemic may strike with consequent increased illness and death for those infected and increased risks to the general population. This has been largely ignored by public health professions and the media. There is growing recognition that TB and HIV programmes need to work together.

Biomedical interventions

The ultimate solution to HIV would be a scientific breakthrough producing a cheap, effective vaccine. Since Edward Jenner vaccinated an 8-year-old boy against smallpox in 1796, vaccines have been the accepted way of eliminating diseases. The first disease to be eradicated worldwide was indeed smallpox—the last 'wild' case occurring in 1977. The world is on the cusp of eradicating polio with only a handful of cases emerging each year.

Unfortunately progress towards a vaccine is slow. In April 1984, when she announced that scientists had identified the virus that caused AIDS, Margaret Heckler also said a vaccine would be 'ready for testing in approximately two years'. Since then, despite the efforts of scientists, only one vaccine has been found, with limited efficacy (this was reported in 2009). It reduced infections by about 31 per cent in Thai military recruits. Other candidate vaccines have, so far, shown no effectiveness, although there were at least twenty trials underway in 2015.

Vaccines are seen as crucial by policymakers, scientists, doctors, and activists. In 1995, treatment activists founded the AIDS Vaccine Advocacy Coalition to speed the development of HIV vaccines. The International AIDS Vaccine Initiative (IAVI) estimates that an effectively rolled-out inoculation programme providing 70 per cent protection could reduce new infections by 40 per cent in the first ten years and by half in twenty-five years.

At the World Economic Forum in Davos in 2015, Bill Gates predicted that there would be an AIDS vaccine by 2030. Even when an effective vaccine is developed, there will be issues of economics and compliance. Vaccine development is resource intensive and, although most research is conducted in the rich world, there is little commercial incentive—the market is limited and risks are high. When a vaccine is developed there will be questions as to what degree of protection it would offer, and for what duration. Would one dose be sufficient, or would boosters be required?

Another option is a 'microbicide'—a substance inserted into the vagina prior to intercourse that will kill viruses and bacteria, providing women with protection they can themselves control. However, development of microbicides has been slow. There was early optimism when a trial in 2010, the CAPRISA 004 trial, showed that tenofovir gel, when applied before and after sex, reduced HIV incidence by 39 per cent. Unfortunately, two subsequent trials have reported no benefits, although it is thought that this is probably because the women were not using the microbicides consistently. There are numerous other trials underway, including one of a rectal microbicide. In time, a microbicide is expected to be added to the armamentarium against HIV but it is uncertain when.

Research into vaccines and microbicides is important but early optimism has given way to a new realism. Both interventions are some years away, and even when they do become available they will only be one part of the response. Money and science will not be enough to provide solutions to the epidemic.

Australian demographers Jack and Pat Caldwell, as early as 1993, suggested links between male circumcision and patterns of HIV infection. The science was clear. In uncircumcised men, the area under the foreskin and the foreskin itself contains the cells the virus binds to (the Langerhans' cells). The skin or mucosal surface of the foreskin is more easily penetrated. Additionally, circumcised men are less likely to contract and pass on other sexually transmitted infections (STIs).

In South Africa, a study at Orange Farm outside Johannesburg suggested circumcision was 60 per cent protective against HIV infection for men. The study was stopped in November 2004 after analysis showed 'the protection effect' of male circumcision was so high that it would have been unethical to continue. Results were confirmed by further randomized controlled trials in Kisumu, Kenya, and Rakai District, Uganda. Indeed the most recent data from Uganda show effectiveness may be higher over time. WHO and UNAIDS recommend voluntary medical male circumcision

(VMMC) as an important prevention intervention, particularly in areas of high HIV prevalence and low levels of circumcision. Fears of 'disinhibition', that is, circumcised men having more sexual partners in the belief that they are protected, have been shown to be unfounded.

Circumcision can be carried out surgically or with medical devices. One such device has been prequalified by the WHO. This means it meets standards of quality, safety, and demonstrated efficacy for international use. Other methods are in development. While access to circumcision should be made available for men and adolescent boys, it is less complicated and risky for infants, so neo-natal circumcision should be promoted. While the criticism that it will take twenty years for the effect to be appreciated is true, had the measure been introduced at the outset, in 1996, the benefits would be evident today.

The role of ART treatment in prevention

In 2011, the HPTN 052 trial reported its findings concerning the level of protection ART provides to the uninfected sexual partners of HIV+ people. The study was conducted in eighteen sites in eight countries. It began enrolling participants in 2005, recruiting 1,736 sero-discordant couples. Most were heterosexual, but 3 per cent were male couples. The study found the efficacy of treatment as prevention to be 96 per cent. HIV+ people taking ARVs were more than twenty times less likely to infect their partners. Effectively, the virus they carry is supressed. This study was supposed to continue to 2015 but it too was stopped for ethical reasons, once the reduction in transmissions became obvious. This has given rise to the argument and advocacy for treatment as prevention or TasP, which was reinforced by the Strategic Timing of Anti-Retroviral Therapy (START) study that took place in 2009 and was reported in 2015. This study was carried out in 215 sites in thirty-five countries, and it concluded that early initiation of ART is beneficial to all HIV-infected individuals.

Drugs have been used for many years by medical staff for post-exposure prophylaxis (PEP). If a person is at risk, most usually due to needle stick injury, ART should be taken as soon as possible. The CDC recommends, for most exposures, a two-drug regimen for four weeks. PEP can also be used for non-occupational exposure such as unprotected sex or sexual assault. There has been recent interest in pre-exposure prophylaxis (PrEP). This involves HIV negative (HIV–) people taking drugs daily to reduce their risk of infection. In early 2016, the use of daily Truvada (a combination of tenofovir and emtricitabine) was approved in the US for MSM and others at risk of sexual transmission. Adherence is crucial and the cost is high ($800 per month in 2016).

In mid-2015, UNAIDS under the leadership of Michel Sidibé, launched the 90–90–90 'fast track' goals for ending the epidemic by 2030: by 2020, 90 per cent of all people living with HIV will know their HIV status; 90 per cent of all people with diagnosed HIV infection will receive sustained antiretroviral therapy; and 90 per cent of all people receiving antiretroviral therapy will have viral suppression. By 2030, these numbers should have risen to 95 per cent for each target. The pros and cons of TasP are discussed in Chapter 7.

The pace of scientific discovery has picked up over the last decade. There has been (admittedly optimistic) talk of a potential cure. Social and behavioural drivers of the epidemic have slipped down the agenda. Unfortunately, despite the recognition in public health that 'an ounce of prevention is worth a pound of cure', this message is still not getting through. While new infections fall the number of infected people continues to rise.

Chapter 3
What shapes epidemics?

Disease, including AIDS, is a sickness of the body. AIDS is the presenting symptom. The manifestations of AIDS, illness, and death reveal the fractures, stresses, and strains in a society. While at the most proximate level, the chance of HIV transmission depends on biological determinants, there are other factors that need to be considered, in particular social and economic poverty and inequality.

The overview of global epidemiology revealed a range of epidemics. Globally HIV prevalence has peaked: in some locations it rose to unexpected levels and remains high; in others (such as Uganda), it declined but numbers are beginning to rise again. There are settings where all the factors that would facilitate HIV spread seem to be in place, yet there is no epidemic. While biomedical factors are critical, it is ultimately behaviours that determine the shape of the epidemic. Social and environmental factors: the position people occupy in society, their economic status, how they are perceived, and how they value themselves all affect risk. Where vulnerabilities converge, the most serious epidemics follow.

If we can explain existing epidemics, can we predict new ones? Where prevalence has fallen, can we understand what happened in order that it can be replicated elsewhere? Why is there a second wave of HIV infections in some countries?

Infections and epidemics don't happen randomly. Some diseases are limited to certain geographical environments—malaria occurs where a specific species of mosquito can live. People have to be exposed to the pathogen. Even then, for an infection to take hold, the immune system must be unable to resist the disease-causing organism. This is true of all infectious illnesses. It is seen each year with the common cold, many are exposed to the virus, but some manage to stave off infection while others fall sick.

Drivers of disease are firstly social and economic. For example, living in poorly ventilated, crowded rooms increases the risk of exposure to and contraction of TB. Those who are undernourished and/or lacking vitamins and micro-nutrients will have increased susceptibility to a plethora of illnesses, and will be sicker for longer.

The importance of the social determinants of health (SDH) has long been recognized. The Whitehall Studies, beginning in 1967, looked at heart disease and mortality in British civil servants. The lowest grades had mortality rates three times higher than those in the highest grades. In 2008 the *WHO Commission on Social Determinants of Health Report* was published and the organization now has an SDH unit. However, AIDS seemed to confound this observation, as initially wealthier people had higher rates of infection.

Nonetheless, disease, globally and nationally, flourishes where there is poverty. In rich countries, the greatest disease burden is among the poorer groups: those who are marginalized, ill-nourished, poorly housed, and less well-educated. With regard to nations, broadly speaking, it is in the poorer ones where disease is more likely to thrive. There are exceptions to this. Critical factors that can mitigate poverty and poor health are proactive social and public health services. Thus Cuba and Kerala State in India have healthier populations than their richer, less equitable neighbours.

On occasion, there is a convergence of vulnerability which results in devastating epidemic outbreaks. Prior to 1991, cholera had not been seen in the Americas for a hundred years. In that year, an outbreak began in Peru after a ship in Lima harbour pumped its bilges of water contaminated by the *Vibrio cholerae* bacteria. The disease took hold in the city's favelas and then spread from slum to slum across the Americas. Obviously ships had previously discharged contaminated water in Lima and elsewhere. However in 1991, the slums had grown rapidly, and the slum dwellers were victims of a decade of economic crisis, with falling incomes and increased inequality. People were poorly nourished and lacked access to basic infrastructure facilities, including running water, sanitation, and health services. The consequence was the region-wide cholera epidemic.

Ebola in West Africa is a second and more recent example. The first recorded outbreak of Ebola was in Southern Sudan in June 1976. There were sporadic occurrences in Central Africa over the subsequent thirty years that were either contained or spluttered out. In March 2014, cases of Ebola were reported in south-western Guinea. Within a few days, Sierra Leone and Liberia notified the WHO that they too were treating patients. The collapse of public health services, rapid urbanization, insanitary slum conditions, and mobility of people all contributed to this. Few cases of Ebola occurred in the rich world and most were 'imported' from West Africa.

Biomedical drivers

In order for a person to become infected, they must be in contact with HIV, with sufficient exposure for the infection to take hold.

Once contact has occurred, biomedical factors are the key determinant of whether or not a person will be infected.

Most important biological drivers relate to the virus sub-type involved, and the health status and genetic makeup of those exposed. Some viral sub-types are more infectious than others. This may partly explain why Southern Africa, where sub-type clade C is found, has such a serious epidemic. Controversially, the genetics of a populace are important, at both an individual and a population level, making some groups more or less susceptible. Sometimes interpreted as a form of putative 'genetic determinism', this reality results from the diverse genetic variance of humankind. Evolution is not 'kind' or 'cruel', although we may wish to construe it as such. The importance of the virus type and the genetics of those infected or not are areas of continued scientific research.

The stage of infection is crucial. For several months after infection there is an intense battle between the immune system and the virus. During this period the semen/vaginal fluids and blood contain many virus particles, which raises the chance of infection for sexual partners and people who share injecting equipment. There is then a period when the body rallies and the viral load is low, decreasing risk of transmission. As the infection progresses the viral load will slowly climb again and the CD4 count will fall, as shown in Figure 5.

Once an epidemic takes hold in a society, it has a built-in momentum. The more people with early-stage infection, the greater the chance of a non-infected person having sex with one of these infected people and being infected. A vicious cycle develops.

The virus has to breach the natural defences of the body: the skin or mucous membranes. Risk is higher for women as semen remains in the vagina after unprotected intercourse. This partly accounts for the greater number of women infected in heterosexually driven epidemics. The danger is increased by tearing in the vagina, which may occur during rape or abusive and rough sex, especially in younger women whose genitalia are not mature. Interventions that delay sexual debut can reduce transmission. Condoms provide a barrier, but are not necessarily female controlled.

STIs are an important biological co-factor. Those that cause genital ulcers, such as herpes, cancroid, and syphilis, create a portal for the virus to enter the body, and at the same time the presence of the cells HIV seeks to infect, CD4 cells and macrophages, is increased. In a person with an STI, the number of virus particles released into blood, semen, and other body fluids increases, even if the infection is asymptomatic. An HIV-infected person is more likely to be infected by STIs, and the severity and duration of these infections will be increased.

After sexual transmission, the next most important route for HIV infection is vertical transmission, when a mother's infection is passed to the child. The viral load of the mother influences the chance of infection—the higher the load, the higher the risk. However, if a woman has advanced disease, her chance of falling pregnant and carrying a child to term is decreased.

Other biomedical drivers include the use of unsafe blood and blood products and nosocomial infections. While 'nosocomial' usually means infections acquired in hospital, with regard to HIV it is taken to mean all infections transmitted in health care settings. If equipment is not adequately sterilized then there is a danger of patient-to-patient transmission. Health workers are at risk through accidents involving body fluids such as needle stick injuries. All those caring for AIDS patients, including in the home, face some slight danger, and this rises if people don't have adequate protective equipment such as gloves. Sharing drug-injecting apparatus is an efficient way of spreading HIV, and is, in some settings, the main driver.

One under-researched area is the effect of ill health on HIV transmission. There is evidence to suggest any infection will cause the viral load to rise rapidly and remain high for some time. For example, when somebody has malaria, the level of virus in the blood increases tenfold and thus such a person will be more infectious to his or her partners. They may not want to have sex while they are sick—however, when they recover, their sex drive will return and infectivity is still high. Researchers in Kisumu, Kenya, estimated that 5 per cent of adult HIV infections were linked to malaria. HIV infection also increases susceptibility to other diseases, the Kenyan research suggested 10 per cent of malaria cases were due to HIV.

Finally, as was discussed in Chapter 2, circumcision in men is a simple and effective biomedical measure in preventing contraction of HIV.

Behaviour

In order for biomedical factors to come into play, a person has to have sex, or share needles, with someone who is infected. There are a range of behaviours that increase risk. The AIDS epidemic has taught us unexpected lessons about human sexuality. For example, the frequency of sexual intercourse does not vary greatly from country to country; there is a diverse and intriguing variety of sexual practices, most of which are harmless and many of which are considered 'normal'; and the behaviours that facilitate the spread of HIV are complex and dynamic. (Box 3.)

If someone does not have sex or keeps to one uninfected partner, then that person won't be sexually exposed to HIV (or any other sexually transmitted infection), provided their partner is also

Box 3 Data on sex and sexuality

We are all intrigued by sex and sexual behaviours, but collecting this information is complex. The first study was by Dr Alfred Kinsey of Indiana University. The Kinsey Reports comprise companion volumes on human sexual behaviour, *Sexual Behavior in the Human Male* (1948) and *Sexual Behavior in the Human Female* (1953). This research was controversial, not just for the subject matter, but because it challenged beliefs about sexuality including the idea that heterosexuality, faithfulness, and abstinence were ethical and statistical norms. Kinsey said. 'We are the recorders and reporters of facts—not the judges of the behaviors we describe.'

A basic problem is data are self-reported and subject to bias. A Tanzanian article on sexuality entitled: 'Secretive Females or Swaggering Males?' found that men over-report and women under-report numbers of partnerships and frequency of intercourse. The 2006 Lancet meta-analysis showed how little data there were on sexual behaviour; and literature searches failed to find more recent quality comparative global information.

faithful. This applies in all sexual relationships, hetero or homosexual. In societies where polygamy is practiced, as long as all are faithful, the same protections apply. Early AIDS prevention posters, which in most countries said, unequivocally, 'Stick to One Partner' had to be adapted for Swaziland where polygamy is accepted and the king has many wives. Here the posters had the less than catchy message: 'Be Faithful in Your Polygamous Family'.

Key behavioural factors are: the age of sexual debut, sexual practices, number of partners, frequency of partner exchange, concurrency, and mixing patterns including intergenerational sex. The younger a woman begins sex, the greater her risk of infection.

The age of sexual debut is determined by her behaviour, that of her partners, and the cultural practices and social norms of her environment. Social dislocation decreases inhibition and increases vulnerability. Globally data suggest females have sex earlier than males, but trends for age-at-first-sex are unclear.

The median age for first sexual intercourse in Zambia in 2013, was 17.3 for females and 18.3 for males; in Mozambique in 2011, 17.1 for females and 16.1 for males. Both countries have serious epidemics. In the Philippines where there was a concern HIV might spread, sexual debut is 21.5 for females and 22.3 for males. In the UK, debut is 16 for both genders and in USA 17 for males and 17.3 for females. However, as shown, health including sexual health is better in the West and also condoms are widely used.

Prevalence of premarital sex increases if marriage is postponed. There is evidence from South Africa that marriage rates are declining: the number of civil marriages fell from 178,689 in 2002 to 167,264 in 2011, while the number of registered customary marriages fell from 17,283 to just 5,084. Population increased from forty-six to fifty-three million in this period. Prevalence in 2012 was 10 per cent for those in a marriage, 24.3 per cent among people 'going steady or living together', and 14.3 per cent among the singles.

The question of which sexual practices are most risky is one that receives more salacious press than is deserved, despite it being the area we know least about in terms of risk of infection. Examples of potentially harmful practices are widow inheritance, where a woman is 'inherited' by her deceased husband's brother; and the practice of 'dry sex', where herbs or other agents are used to dry out the vagina, which some believe increases (the man's) pleasure during sex. The range of practices is immense. It is necessary to be open-minded in discussing these in order to facilitate identifying those which increase risk, how they do this, and what can be done to decrease the likelihood of transmission.

The number of sexual partners per se seems less important. Men in Thailand (where the adult infection rate is 1.1 per cent) and Rio de Janeiro (adult infection rate in Brazil 0.5 per cent) were more likely to report five or more casual partners in the previous year than men in Tanzania and Lesotho. However, in these African countries adult infection rates were 5.3 per cent and 23.4 per cent, respectively. The HSRC's 2012 South African study found 37.5 per cent of males and 8.2 per cent of females aged 15–24 reported having more than one partner in the preceding twelve months; yet the corresponding prevalence rates are 2.9 per cent and 11.4 per cent, showing the gendered nature of risk.

People in industrialized countries do not have significantly more or fewer partners in a lifetime than those in other parts of the world, although their tendency is for serial monogamy. This means that they enter relationships which are maintained for months or years. The relationships involve a degree of commitment, and may be legally recognized as marriage or civil union. Serial monogamy traps the virus within a single relationship, reducing the risk for HIV transmission. The danger of infection increases when people have 'non-regular' partners or affairs.

While frequent partner change is hazardous, it is not common anywhere. The greater risk is believed to be concurrency of partnering, when people have more than one partner and the relationships overlap. Writing in the *Lancet* in 2004 Halperin and Epstein noted, because infectivity is higher during the period after infection, this sexual practice of concurrency greatly exacerbates the spread of HIV. When one person in a network of concurrent relationships becomes infected, everyone is at risk.

Commercial sex which includes both heterosexual and homosexual transactions is also potentially risky for sex workers and their partners. In many settings in the early years of the epidemic, commercial sex workers were 'core transmitters'. A modelling exercise in Nairobi illustrated this. It assumed that

80 per cent of sex workers were infected and had four partners per day; and that 10 per cent of men were infected and had four partners per year. Increasing condom use from 10 per cent to 80 per cent by commercial sex workers was estimated to prevent 10,200 new infections. On the other hand increasing condom use among the men to 80 per cent would only avert eighty-eight infections. In Thailand, the initial epidemic was spread by sex workers, but the '100% condom campaign', making condom use mandatory in brothels, brought HIV under control.

Mixing patterns facilitates infection spread from one part of a country to another, and across national borders. Here paths for transmission include both sex and drug use. For example, an oil worker who becomes infected in, say, Nigeria can carry the disease to his or her home country, then to, say, Indonesia in a matter of days. A Central Asian drug user can fly to any European capital in hours. With this there is the danger of re-infection and of new strains evolving.

Mixing not only takes place across geographic regions but also across age groups. Intergenerational sex, usually where men have younger female partners, is common in many societies. In countries where there is a heterosexual epidemic, women in their teens and twenties have higher prevalence than their male peer group, as shown in the HSRC data on Figure 3. This is because they are having sex with older infected men, and it may be transactional: for money, clothes, food, transport, or school and university fees.

The use of condoms is also a 'behaviour'. Correct, consistent condom use reduces the chance of HIV infection. Where condoms were used in risky settings—among young people in Europe and the United States, and in brothels in Thailand—they prevented HIV spread or they turned the epidemic around. It is, however, difficult to achieve consistent use, other than in commercial and casual sexual encounters. Women may not have the power to insist their partners use condoms and in long-term relationships it is hard to sustain condom use.

Social, economic, political, and other determinants

How people behave may determine their risk of infection, but behaviours result from the environment in which people live and operate. This milieu is, in turn, a function of local, national, and international factors: economics, politics, and culture. These are complex and varied, and how we view them depends on our own values, backgrounds, and disciplines. How the epidemic is influenced by these determinants is best illustrated by examples.

In Southern Africa, development of mines and industry required large quantities of labour. The dominance of capitalism meant wages were tightly controlled. The colonial history and, in South Africa, subsequent Apartheid legislation, resulted in black labour being most exploited. Apartheid imposed strict controls on where black people could live and work. Huge numbers of men travelled for employment in the mines, factories, and on the farms. Foreign migrant miners drawn primarily from Malawi, Lesotho, Botswana, Swaziland, Mozambique, and Namibia worked on contracts in South Africa. In 1985 nearly two million black South Africans were classified as migrants, effectively foreigners in their own country. These people lived apart from their families, mostly in crowded, single-sex hostels, and were forced to return home between contracts.

The effects of this dislocation and disempowerment have been well-documented. When people are put in circumstances where they cannot maintain stable relationships—where life is risky, and pleasures are few and necessarily cheap—then sexually transmitted diseases will be rampant. This was true for all migrants. For migrant miners their work was more dangerous, their control over most aspects of their lives was minimal, and they were disempowered in many respects. However they had regular incomes. When this was factored in with the gender inequality and extreme poverty in the surrounding communities, an ideal setting had been created for the spread of STIs.

During the 1980s, four large surveys were carried out to establish if HIV was present in South African populations. It was not found. However the mines identified it in a few Malawian miners. Migration created the perfect environment for the spread of HIV, not only in labour-using centres but in the migrants' home communities. The fracturing of families, changing gender dynamics, and increased poverty drove the epidemic. Decades after the end of Apartheid, the migrant labour system has shrunk. At the peak in 1977 there were over 577,000 migrants on contract to the mines. In 1990 as HIV began to spread, there were still about 375,000; in 2015 there were fewer than 250,000, but the damage had already been done in the 1990s.

Similar stories can be told of former communist countries. The collapse of communism was not good news for millions of citizens of the Soviet Union and Eastern Bloc. The old regime provided many benefits: people were assured of employment, education, housing, health care, and even holidays. Basic needs, and more, were met. The breakdown of these economies has been well-documented. In the Ukraine the per capita GDP fell from US$6,372 in 1990 to a low of US$3,194 in 1998. The number of unemployed reached close to three million by 2000: 12 per cent of the economically active population. Alcohol abuse was always common, but intravenous drug use increased dramatically, especially among the dispossessed and lost youth. The epidemic was driven by drug use, which in turn was the result of economic and social disintegration, and the consequent blow to the morale, hopes, and dreams of the younger generation.

Gender relations shape risk and behaviours. A woman's biology puts her at greater risk. Of crucial importance is womens' lack of power and the violence against them. Girls often feel pressured or are forced into having sex. South Africa's Medical Research Council reported in 2009 that one in four South African men admitted to having 'had sex with a woman when she didn't consent', and 46 per cent of those said they had done so more than once. The rate of rape per 100,000 according to United Nations Office on Drugs and Crime (UNODC) was 90.6 in Lesotho and 29.6 in Jamaica. The WHO notes that violence against women is a major public health problem, 35 per cent of women worldwide have experienced either intimate-partner violence or non-partner sexual violence in their lives. Physically or sexually abused women were 1.5 times more likely to have an STI compared to women who had not experienced partner violence.

Some customs encourage early marriage and pregnancy; the marriage of young women to older men; and unequal partnering. These promote male dominance and female subservience. Globally social norms emphasize female chastity and turn a blind eye to male promiscuity. In much of the poor world, women are economically dependent on men, and sex work is an extreme manifestation. Enabling female control of reproductive health would be an HIV and AIDS intervention.

The relationship between HIV and AIDS and poverty is complex, at both an individual and a national level. Botswana is a wealthy African country, with a per capita GDP of US$7,123 in 2014, the fifth highest in sub-Saharan Africa; Senegal by contrast has a GDP of just US$1,061 per capita. The adult prevalence rates are 25.2 per cent in Botswana and 0.5 per cent in Senegal. Simply being a poor country does not mean higher HIV prevalence. What seems crucial is equality within the nation. At the individual level data are also unclear. Demographic and health survey (DHS) data from Burkina Faso, Cameroon, Ghana, Kenya, Lesotho, Malawi, Tanzania, and Uganda show that, contrary to evidence for other infectious diseases and intuitive expectations, HIV prevalence is not disproportionately high among poorer adults in sub-Saharan Africa.

The big picture

While, at that the most proximate level, the chance of HIV transmission may depend on biological determinants, they are only a part of the picture. Developing drugs, vaccines, and microbicides, circumcising men, and putting people on treatment are effective technical and biomedical responses. Unfortunately this disease does not lend itself to simple technical solutions. The real challenge is to reduce risk. Behaviours can be modified. The evidence suggests that there are a few key interventions which would have a significant impact on the progress of the epidemic: reducing concurrent partnering and delaying sexual debut, for example. Beyond this are the messages used since the early days: abstinence, fidelity, and condom use.

Both behaviours and biomedical factors are determined by how a society operates at the macro level: its culture, politics, and economics. These are crucial, and most important are gender relations and income equality. The central issue is how people view and treat one another. A society in which people respect the views and choices of others is one in which unsafe sex is less likely to occur.

Preventing HIV transmission requires a greater understanding of the determinants. Unfortunately for those currently infected, those who have died, and their families and communities, prevention has not worked. We need to understand how AIDS and its consequences will evolve through society and what the role of treatment might be.

Chapter 4
Illness, death, and the demographic impact

Prior to the introduction of ART, an HIV infection led to illness and eventual death. The consequences of AIDS stem from this increased morbidity and mortality. Treatment means that if a person is able to access the drugs and is adherent, illness and death can be avoided, or at least postponed. In the case of infants, whose infection stems from vertical transmission, prevention is straightforward provided they and their mothers are reached.

Demography and the epidemic

Demography is the study of population dynamics. It collects data on quantifiable events for analysis and projection. The basic data sources are censuses, civil registration, collection of vital statistics, in some countries demographic and health surveys (DHSs), and household surveys. Most censuses are undertaken every ten years, so other data sources are invaluable, especially since the release of census data may take years. Demographers and planners want to know, at a minimum, the number of births, fertility and death rates, and migration patterns.

An increasingly important source of information is civil registration, defined by the United Nations as the 'Universal, continuous, permanent and compulsory recording of vital events'. This recording of milestones including birth, marriage, divorce, adoption, and death is a government responsibility. The process provides individuals with documents to secure recognition of their identity, family relationships, nationality, social protection, and inheritance. It facilitates access to essential services: health, education, and welfare; is important for political engagement (voting); and economic activity (bank accounts and employment).

Vital statistics and the ability to monitor and respond to causes of death and disability underpin national and international targets, including the sustainable development goals (SDGs), universal health coverage, and tackling epidemics. In South Africa birth registrations rose from fewer than 25 per cent in 1991 to over 90 per cent in 2012. Similar improvements have been recorded in death registration, which is compulsory before legal burial or cremation. It allowed deaths to be tracked and AIDS impact inferred.

Demographic consequences of AIDS may include: increased deaths especially among adults; rising infant and child mortality; falling life expectancy; changes in the population size, growth, and structure; and growing numbers of orphans. How serious these impacts are depends on the location, size, and age of the epidemic; the underlying demographics of a country; and, increasingly, the availability and uptake of treatment.

Increased mortality in adults

In the USA, prior to ART, AIDS was the leading cause of mortality for young men, killing some 21,000 in 1995. In 2013 AIDS was ranked as the seventh most important cause of mortality for males in this age group, accounting for 8,324 deaths. The African American community bears a disproportionate burden with 6,540 deaths.

In most countries the number of deaths has peaked. In Uganda the highest level of mortality was in the 1990s. As a result many children were orphaned. While grandparents (especially grandmothers), older siblings, and the community generally ensured these children had some support, most were materially deprived and all bear emotional scars. They are the young adults and, increasingly, the parents of today.

The increase in deaths was the most visible and measurable effect of AIDS. In Southern Africa, prevalence rates rose rapidly from 1992, and in the early part of the new millennium there was a quantifiable and significant rise in deaths. This was dramatically illustrated by data from South Africa's vital registration system. In 2001 the Medical Research Council released a report analysing registered deaths. It showed mortality had shifted from the old to the young, particularly to young women, and there was differential mortality by gender. The future burden of the epidemic was predictable in terms of deaths if treatment was not made available, and in numbers needing treatment if it was.

This was the time South Africa was entering its 'denial period'. President Thabo Mbeki argued, confusedly, that HIV did not exist, but if it did then it was not a killer virus. He was backed by Minister of Health Manto Tsabalala-Msimang, who became known as Dr Beetroot for her advocacy that people eat garlic, beetroot, and lemon to stay healthy. The attitudes were greeted with disbelief by most scientists and health professionals, and some senior government and political figures. It was partly resolved when Mbeki announced he was withdrawing from the discussion, and from 2004 the public health service in South Africa began rolling out ART. University of Cape Town economist Nicoli Nattrass estimated there were more than 340,000 unnecessary AIDS deaths between 1999 and 2007 as a result of this policy.

The changing mortality is shown in Figure 6. Deaths among women aged 30 to 34 more than quadrupled between 1997 and 2005, from 7,196 to 31,283, and then fell to just under 14,000 in

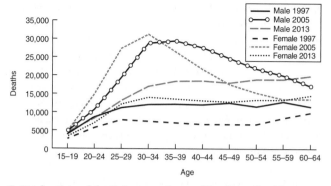

6. Total registered deaths by age and year of death, South Africa.

2013. Among men the peak in mortality was slightly later, but with the same change in the pattern and numbers. The cause of death is not ascribed in the data: the graphs simply show numbers. However, *caeteris paribus*, it is clear AIDS mortality and subsequent availability of treatment is at the root of changing configurations.

The earliest and gloomiest projections of the likely effects of AIDS came from the US Bureau of the Census. Their 2004 report, 'The AIDS Pandemic in the 21st Century', produced country data 'with AIDS' and 'without AIDS'. The figures were bleak. In Botswana, in 2002, the crude death rate (CDR)—the deaths per 1,000 people— was estimated at 28.6, without AIDS it could have been a mere 4.8. Data from the WHO Global Health Observatory gives Botswana's 2013 CDR as 7.2. For Tanzania the 2002 figures were: without AIDS 12.1, with AIDS 17.3; the 2013 figure is 7.8. The top CDR in a high prevalence country is Lesotho's 14.1 in 2013.

Infant and child mortality

Infant and child mortality rose, due partly to vertical transmission. Intervention can eliminate this: it is rare for infants in the developed world to be born with or acquire HIV infection. In some of the poor world preventing vertical transmission remains challenging. In 2014, globally 220,000 children were newly infected, however UNAIDS says in twenty-one priority African countries 77 per cent of pregnant women received ART, and the number of infant infections fell by 48 per cent between 2009 and 2014. The 2014 Swaziland Multiple Indicator Cluster Survey (SMICS) found 95.3 per cent of women reporting a live birth in the last two years were offered and accepted an HIV test, and received the results.

Infected infants have poor life expectancy. In the developed world 70 per cent of those infected at birth are alive at 6 years and 50 per cent at 9 years. In the poor world progression rates are faster. About 25 per cent of HIV infected babies develop symptoms of AIDS or die within the first year. Treating children is a growing global priority but drug development lags, perhaps because transmission can be eliminated and there are not the same profits to be made from paediatric medicines.

The second reason for increased under-5 mortality is deaths among infected mothers. Losing a mother for any reason has an adverse impact on child survival. A 2004 review of the demographic and socio-economic impact of AIDS in the journal *AIDS* noted that the death of a mother increased the chance of a child dying by three times in the year before the mother's death, and by five times in the year after it. Increased child mortality was not affected by the mother's cause of death, but HIV-infected mothers are much more likely to die.

The child mortality rate (CMR), which is the death of a child between 1 and 5, illustrates both the impact of the disease and the roll-out of treatment. The World Bank database provides figures as shown in Table 4. It can be seen that CMR falls with development, rises with the arrival of the epidemic, and then falls again as treatment becomes available.

Table 4 Changing child mortality rates in selected countries

Country (year of independence)	CMR at independence	Lowest CMR post-independence	Highest CMR post-independence	CMR in 2015
Botswana (1966)	139.5	53 (1988)	82.9 (2000)	43.6
Lesotho (1966)	188.5	87.9 (1991)	123.4 (2005)	90.2
South Africa (1994)	133.4 (1974 data)	58.4 (1992)	78.1 (2003)	40.5
Swaziland (1968)	183.5	74.7 (1990)	133.7 (2003)	60.7

The World Bank: Mortality rate, under-5 (per 1,000 live births). http://data.worldbank.org/indicator/SH.DYN.MORT

Falling life expectancy

The effect of AIDS on life expectancy was dramatic in Southern
and Eastern Africa. There was a small impact in Thailand and it
was negligible elsewhere.

Data for selected African countries are shown in Figure 7. The
first country to track a fall in life expectancy was Uganda in
the mid-1980s, albeit from a low level. The shocking lack of
improvement in life expectancy in the post-independence period
was due to the coup that brought dictator Idi Amin to power in
1971; the seven-year political turmoil that followed his overthrow
in 1979, up to 1986; and the subsequent war when current
president Yoweri Museveni swept to power, bringing stability to
Uganda. This political and economic mayhem contributed to the
spread of HIV and AIDS, and continued to erode life expectancy
in the early years of Museveni's rule. However he was also the first
African leader to respond to the epidemic: life expectancy was
turned around and continues to rise.

Botswana's life expectancy was age 52 at independence in 1966;
after twenty-five years of stable political rule and steady economic
growth it was 63. In 1991, AIDS mortality began climbing. By
2006, forty years after independence, life expectancy was just
46, although it is recovering. The lowest life expectancy recorded
in a high prevalence country was age 43 in 2001 in Zimbabwe.
Obviously the political and economic turmoil under the
malevolent rule of Robert Mugabe contributed to this. The
graph shows Zimbabwe to be an outlier since life expectancy
is almost back to the pre-AIDS level, a possible example of
dubious data.

The data do not show what this catastrophic decline in life
expectancy actually means. Did it affect societal ability to
function? This issue is returned to, but it is worth stressing that

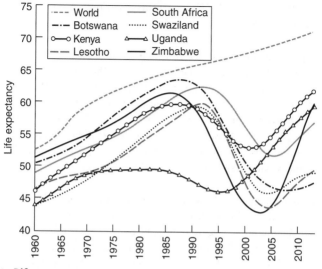

7. **Life expectancy.**

we do not know, partly because impacts are still evolving;
demographers don't think in these terms; and most other social
scientists are not engaged.

Changing population composition

Increased numbers of deaths reduce population growth and
size. Some 1.2 million, mostly young adults, died from AIDS in
2014. In the worst-affected countries the mortality is still
considerable: Statistics South Africa reports that in 2014 there
were 171,733 AIDS deaths in South Africa, down from a peak of
363,910 recorded in 2005; UNAIDS data record 170,000 deaths
in Nigeria in 2014, up from 130,000 in 2000. Outside Africa the
greatest mortality is in Indonesia where 34,000 people died
in 2014; in 2000 there were fewer than 1,000 deaths. In
Thailand the number of deaths fell from 54,000 to 19,000

over the same period. Ukraine saw deaths increase from 6,300 to 15,000.

Population growth decreases due to premature death, reduced fertility, and changing sexual behaviours. As the epidemic progresses there are fewer women of childbearing age. HIV+ women are less likely to conceive and carry the infant to term, thus further reducing the number of live births. Behaviour change has significant potential effects. Condoms now used to protect against disease also have an impact on fertility. A higher age of sexual debut will reduce the total fertility rate.

In most countries AIDS simply means the population will grow more slowly. In India and China the impact is small as the populations are so large and the epidemic relatively insignificant. The UN estimated that in China, in 2015, the population was only 0.16 per cent lower due to AIDS. In Southern and parts of Eastern Africa AIDS has, according to UN data, lead to smaller populations—as shown in Table 5—with consequent potential impacts for economies and social services.

In Eastern Europe, AIDS exacerbates troubling economic and demographic situations, with very low fertility rates and declining populations. Births in Russia in November 2014 were down by more than 5 per cent year-on-year, and immigration decreased by more than 10 per cent. Between 1993 and 2015, Russia's population decreased from about 149 to 144 million people. Based on the present trends there could be between 100 and 107 million in 2050. Russia had between 850,000 and 1,300,000 people aged over 15 living with AIDS in 2013. Mortality among the 15- to 30-year-old age group is increasing, and slow treatment roll-out worsens this.

Population pyramids are shown in Figure 8. The first bleak one produced in 2004 by the US Bureau of the Census is the projected impact for Botswana in 2020. The outer bars show the shape and

Table 5 Populations in 2015 with and without AIDS (in thousands)

Country	With AIDS	Without AIDS	Difference	Life expectancy (2013)
South Africa	51,684	57,932	6,248	57
Nigeria	175,928	180,914	4,986	52
Tanzania	52,109	55,362	3,253	61
Uganda	39,710	43,341	3,631	59
Zimbabwe	14,029	17,131	3,102	60
Swaziland	1,287	1,485	198	49
India	1,294,192	1,300,054	5,862	66
Ukraine	44,165	44,496	331	71
Haiti	10,957	11,166	209	63

United Nations, Department of Economic and Social Affairs, Population Division (2010). Population and HIV/AIDS: 2010. Wall chart (United Nations publication, Sales No. E.10.XIII.9)

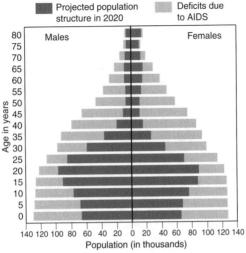

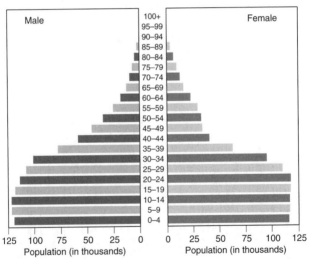

8. Botswana population pyramid with and without AIDS, and 2014 actual.

size of the population in the absence of AIDS. While the gaps in the under-25 age group are a combination of mortality and births that did not occur, among the over-25 age group the change is due to deaths. The second is from 2014. It is clear changing behaviour and the roll-out of ART had a huge effect, although increased mortality can be seen in the 40- to 70-year-old cohorts.

The dependency ratio is an age–population ratio of those not in the labour force (the dependent part including children, people in education, and over-retirement age) and those of working age (the productive part). Conventional dependency ratio calculations assume most adults are productive. In generalized AIDS epidemics, where there is no treatment, significant numbers may be chronically sick and properly belong in the 'dependents' category.

The availability of treatment means social and demographic consequences can be postponed as long as drugs are available and people take them. Providing treatment means population pyramids and dependency ratios won't see the dramatic changes predicted fifteen years ago. Of course, in most of the resource-poor world, the cost of drugs puts them beyond the reach of individuals. They are provided by governments, NGOs, or faith-based organizations. Most funds come from national budgets and/or donors. It is evident therefore that there is a new dependency, of individuals on those who deliver the treatment, and of some nations on international agencies and philanthropic governments.

There may be changes in the gender balance. In heterosexually driven epidemics more women than men are infected and at younger ages. This may influence men to seek sexual relationships with younger and younger women, potentially increasing HIV infection rates. On the other hand, evidence suggests that women are more likely to seek care and therefore get treatment. Where AIDS mortality is high families are held together by the elderly, usually grandmothers.

Orphaning

In classic terms, an orphan is a child who has lost both parents. The definition of 'an orphan' has changed, in large part due to AIDS. The current definition used by UNICEF, other international agencies, and most NGOs for an orphan, is a child under the age of 18, who has lost one or both parents. Maternal orphans have lost a mother, paternal orphans a father, and double orphans both parents.

Globally, in 2012, there were an estimated 150 million orphans, 17.8 million due to AIDS. In sub-Saharan Africa there were fifty-six million orphans of whom 15.1 million were AIDS orphans. Table 6 shows the countries with the largest numbers of AIDS orphans. There are no country data outside Africa.

There are limits to demography. AIDS orphans have different experiences and bear additional burdens compared to those orphaned by other causes. AIDS deaths are protracted. Children who have lost one parent to AIDS risk losing the other, since unprotected heterosexual sex is the major HIV transmission route.

There is an emotional impact which goes uncounted. These children experience many negative changes and can suffer neglect, including emotional abandonment, long before they are orphaned. Death of a parent results in trauma, but AIDS deaths leads to higher levels of psychological distress. Anxiety, depression, and anger are more common among AIDS orphans: 12 per cent of AIDS orphans said 'they wished they were dead': among other orphans the figure was 3 per cent.

Children separated from their siblings can face psychological problems. A 2002 survey in Zambia found more than half of orphans no longer lived with all of their siblings. In Lusaka in

Table 6 Orphaning in selected African countries

Country	Number of children who have lost one or both parents due to all causes	Number of children who have lost one or both parents due to AIDS	Children orphaned by AIDS as a percentage of all orphans
South Africa	4,000,000	2,500,000	63
Nigeria	11,500,000	2,200,000	19
Tanzania	3,100,000	1,200,000	39
Uganda	2,700,000	1,000,000	37
Zimbabwe	1,200,000	890,000	74
Swaziland	120,000	78,000	65

Sources: South Africa (http://www.dhsprogram.com/pubs/pdf/FR206/FR206.pdf); Nigeria (http://www.dhsprogram.com/pubs/pdf/FR293/FR293.pdf); Tanzania (http://www.dhsprogram.com/pubs/pdf/FR243/FR243%5B24June2011%5D.pdf); Uganda (http://www.dhsprogram.com/pubs/pdf/FR264/FR264.pdf); Zimbabwe (http://www.dhsprogram.com/pubs/pdf/FR254/FR254.pdf); Swaziland (http://www.dhsprogram.com/pubs/pdf/FR202/FR202.pdf)

2005, I heard the story of how a grandmother and her sister had taken in two grandchildren, boys aged 9 and 13, when their mother died. Both went to homes with an income, care, and love. One child was taken to the north, the Copperbelt, the other to Livingstone in the south. The women remarked the boys really missed each other and were overjoyed to see each other on the infrequent occasions they met.

Losing a parent to AIDS can have serious consequences for a child's access to basic necessities and education. Orphans are more likely than non-orphans to live in large, female-headed households where more people are dependent on fewer income earners, or with grandparents where there may be no income at all. In her seminal book on HIV and East Africa, reflecting on thirty years of the epidemic, Janet Seeley shows how all too often it is grandparents who bear the burden, usually without support or thanks.

May Chazan's ethnographic study of grandmothers in KwaZulu-Natal has similar findings. Chazan specifically asked Southern African grandmothers why they continued to care for children who they felt were abusive and not committed to their families. One replied, 'We stay here because we love our families, we love the children, and it is our job to raise them'. It is tragic for children to lose parents and tough for the elderly to have to take on unexpected burdens when they are poor and often in ill health. Extended families may absorb orphans, but their capacity and capability is limited.

Children grieving for dying or dead parents may be stigmatized by society through association with AIDS, which leads to shame, fear, and rejection. They may be denied access to schooling and health care because it is assumed that they are infected. Realization of the potential effect of AIDS led to much research, and to many NGOs and especially UNICEF taking steps to proactively address this.

Under my directorship, the Health Economics and HIV/AIDS Research Division (HEARD) carried out two major studies on children affected by illness. The Amajuba Child Health and Wellbeing Research Project conducted in KwaZulu-Natal between 2003 and 2007 found differences between orphan and non-orphan caregivers; the former being more likely to care for more children, have poorer health, experience higher levels of chronic illness, receive less adult help, and bear more daily responsibilities. More orphan caregivers said children in their care needed help for mental or behavioural issues. However only 3.4 per cent of households had contact with child welfare agencies. The second study, with Oxford University in Northern KwaZulu-Natal, examined the impact of living in an AIDS-affected family on the health of children; unsurprisingly it was worse. It found 49 per cent of the caregivers sampled experienced anxiety—considerably higher than the 16 per cent estimated nationally.

Beyond demographics to social and economic impact

At the root of the difficulties in understanding the effects of the epidemic is what we measure, and when and how we measure it. Demography looks at events. An AIDS death is an event. The preceding period of illness is prolonged and debilitating for the individual, and costly and demoralizing for families, households, and communities, but is part of a process and not measured by demographers. The studies carried out by HEARD, Seeley, and others show people cope because there is no other option.

Impacts continue to be felt by families and communities after death. There is evidence that AIDS deaths have more serious consequences for survivors than deaths from other causes. The 'post-death' consequences are not measured by demography. This needs examination by other disciplines. Our work on orphans measured the impact of AIDS; we did less well in changing policy to support children.

The advent of mass treatment has been a game changer. It means deaths can be averted, but at a cost. While the demographic impact may be reduced, the ideas of dependency and dependency rates needs to be reconsidered. People and nations are experiencing a new dependency on the largess of those who provide treatment.

Chapter 5
Production and people

Tracking the social and economic impact of AIDS is more complex than measuring demographic consequences. The epidemic does not have a long history and what we measure is what has, not what will, happen. The research may not ask the right questions or look in right places. There is tension between intensive ethnographic research at an individual level, and national survey instruments that lose this detail. Finally, unsurprisingly, people, communities, and economies have coping strategies. The presence of AIDS means adaptations occur. As a result some predictions were simply wrong; for example the erroneous forecast of 'feral bands of AIDS orphans roaming the streets'.

The conundrum of macro-economic effects

Trying to ascribe causality to HIV and AIDS for economic impact is problematic. There are many other factors to be considered, for example: the price of oil and other commodities; national fiscal policy; and exchange rates. Conventional economics misses the complexity and full significance of the epidemic.

AIDS cannot be treated as an 'exogenous' influence that can be 'tacked on'. In many settings AIDS is a reality, there is no 'without AIDS' scenario. Does AIDS have macro-economic effects? Do these macro-economic impacts in turn have a bearing on the spread of HIV? Do the potential economic impacts slow growth and create development challenges? And does this whole process create a cycle? The potential of these consequences, and possible feedback loops, gave rise to some of the early advocacy that called for the allocation of resources to the epidemic. Do economic returns to investments in HIV and AIDS response magnify the positive impacts of these investments; help build political support; and contribute to refinancing some of the costs of the HIV/AIDS response? The answers to these questions were not entirely clear, which made the task of advocates difficult.

Growth is determined by capital accumulation (both physical and human) and total factor productivity (TFP). TFP is the variable which accounts for output not caused by inputs of labour and capital. AIDS is assumed to affect growth through reduced savings and investment, by cutting the size of the labour force, and by causing efficiency and productivity losses.

Physical capital accumulation happens through savings and investment. AIDS affects this at the individual, company, and international level. For instance, families affected by AIDS deplete their savings and assets in order to cope with increased expenditure and income shocks. Similarly, firm profits (and hence saving and investment) may decrease due to lower labour productivity and increased AIDS-related expenditure. Productivity losses arise directly as HIV and AIDS may affect the output of people living with HIV. High mortality may destroy human capital and deter investments in education and skills.

The models produced in the early 1990s predicted a negative relationship between HIV/AIDS and growth. World Bank economists estimated a 1.2 per cent point reduction in annual growth for a 20 per cent prevalence rate. However, AIDS does not appear to have held back economic growth in Uganda, Botswana, or South Africa. Uganda, with the worst epidemic in the world at the beginning of the 1990s, managed consistent economic progress: GDP growth was estimated at 7 per cent per annum from 1990 to 2000 and 7.7 per cent from 2000 to 2010. Botswana's growth rate over the same period was 5.7 per cent and 4.1 per cent, respectively. South Africa's growth was 2.1 per cent in the 1990s, a time of political turmoil and transition, and then rose to 3.9 per cent from 2000 to 2010, despite the fact that the AIDS morbidity and mortality began to bite at that time. And in the four years from 2010 to 2014 it has averaged 2.44 per cent—yet people are increasingly on treatment.

There is the vexing question of per capita income. This is calculated by dividing the total output of the country by the number of people, usually expressed in US dollars and adjusted for what the dollars will buy in the country: the purchasing power parity. Thus, according to IMF 2014 data, the per capita income in Qatar, the world's richest country, is US$137,162 while the lowest, Central African Republic, is US$607. The per capita incomes in the UK and USA are US$39,826 and US$54,370, respectively. If the people who die are contributing little and their deaths are not affecting overall production then, *in economic terms*, the per capita income may go up. This economic reality is uncomfortable and rarely talked about as it places different values on lives. It also points to the limitations of GDP measures.

If the epidemic is located among the poor or very poor countries, the impact may be minimal. Where peasant farmers' contribution to the formal economy is unimportant and they expect little from the state then their disappearance may be *economically* and *politically* insignificant. In a society with high unemployment among the unskilled, losing people will not have the same economic impact as when there is a skills shortage and the loss is among the skilled.

So what are we to conclude about the macro-economic impact of this disease? Why do the models of AIDS impact and the data appear at odds? Might these countries have grown faster in the absence of AIDS? It is possible that the epidemic may be contributing to South Africa's recent miserable economic performance or Zimbabwe's near collapse, but this is difficult to assess. In his 2016 book *Economics of the Global Response to HIV/ AIDS*, Markus Haacker carries out an exhaustive analysis looking for empirical evidence for the impact of AIDS on economic growth. He concludes: 'it presents an incoherent picture'.

The most we can say is countries (and people) would be better off not experiencing AIDS, but the extent is not clear in macro-economic terms. It does however have implications for advocacy. Ministers of finance are not stupid: arguments about macro-economic effects of HIV and AIDS are weak. New thinking, supported by the RUSH Foundation, looks at 'moral duty'. The researchers led by Oxford economist Sir Paul Collier postulate that given the cost of maintaining lives is so low—a few hundred dollars annually—there is a moral duty to rescue those infected.

To quote (emphasis mine):

> we construct a model to show that in some countries expenditure on prevention would be cost-effective, reducing liabilities by more than its cost. In principle, *prevention should be pursued at least up to the point at which expenditure on it reduces the quasi-liability* sufficiently to minimize the overall cost of accepting the duty to rescue. However...the *quasi-liability is likely to remain too high to be affordable for a significant number of African countries*....if the international community accepts part of the quasi-liability (as it does), it should finance an equal share of prevention and treatment efforts.

AIDS and the private sector

The impact of AIDS on the private sector will depend on the scale of the epidemic in the country or area, the capital/labour mix of the firm, the role of the government in terms of regulation and sharing the burden of AIDS, and what actions individual companies can and do take to avert the effects of the epidemic.

In some countries, firms are experiencing increased illness and death among workers which results in rising costs and falling productivity. AIDS increases the cost of doing business. In Zimbabwe there is the AIDS levy which was introduced in 2000. This requires employed persons and companies to pay 3 per cent of their taxable income towards HIV and AIDS interventions.

More complex is decreased productivity of the workforce due to illness. This is hard to measure except where workers are paid according to output. The first such study by Boston University's Centre for International Health and Development (CIHD) looked at a tea plantation in Kenya where workers were paid per kilogram (kg) of leaf plucked. The CIHD research reviewed records of output and absenteeism from January 1997 to December 2002. HIV-infected individuals plucked on average 3.6 kg/day less tea in the two to three years of the study compared to non-infected employees, and 5.1 kg/day less in the year prior to their death. Their output was 9.3 kg/day less when approaching death.

The question of what happens after initiation of treatment is deeply interesting. In 2006 and 2007 the BU team enrolled tea pluckers who had been initiated on ART, and examined their days worked; kg plucked; and income. The study found that productivity, and hence income, of infected workers decreased significantly before and immediately after initiating ART, but once they were established on the medication it recovered. Men were 90 per cent and women 80 per cent as productive as uninfected co-workers.

Absenteeism and taking of sick leave is easier to record. In Kenya the CIHD study found prior to ART being available, in the three years leading up to death, HIV+ workers used between 3.4 and

11.0 more days of sick leave than uninfected employees, depending on the stage of illness. I (along with others at HEARD) documented similar patterns in a range of other workplaces ranging from cement works to diamond mines and textile mills across Southern Africa. Introduction of treatment 'normalizes' attendance.

Firms are not helpless in the face of the epidemic. They have a range of responses open to them—from changing workforce composition to reducing the benefits. They may, before becoming established in a country, assess the investment climate including the health and skills of the potential employees. In the most extreme cases, they could, if they are footloose (not dependent on local resources), relocate to places with lower HIV prevalence. AIDS can be factored in like any other business cost or threat.

The private sector has a range of options for dealing with HIV, from prevention to treatment of workers. Before public sector treatment programmes became widely available, a number of mainly multinational companies introduced treatment for workers and families. Today HIV is included in broader wellness programmes. What is less clear is how the epidemic affects the environment in which companies operate. The impacts, including decreasing productivity, are often exacerbated in the public sector when compared to the private sector. In the public sector, job security and benefits are a substitute for salary and there is limited capacity to respond. The costs of public sector benefits are borne by government. The costs of declining efficiency are borne by society at large.

It is telling how the importance of AIDS has declined. Private sector organizations that previously focused on AIDS have redefined their mandates. The Global Business Coalition on HIV/AIDS established in 2001, initially by seventeen companies, subsequently became Global Business Coalition on HIV/AIDS, Tuberculosis and Malaria. In June 2011 it rebranded as GBCHealth, with the goal of helping the global business community to fully contribute 'assets, skills, influence and reach to make the world healthier', and to serve as a hub on global health issues. In 2015 it had over 220 companies and organizations as members and affiliates, from all over the world and virtually every industry. The South African Business Coalition on HIV and AIDS (SABCOHA) was established in 2004 'to mobilize and empower business in South Africa to take effective action on HIV and AIDS in the workplace and beyond'. It too has broadened its mandate to all matters relating to health. It neatly changed the H for HIV into an H for Health ensuring the acronym remained the same.

Parts of the private sector have done well out of the epidemic. Most obvious are the pharmaceutical companies that are developing, manufacturing, and supplying drugs. Originally sold at obscenely high prices, pressure from activists and others brought the costs down dramatically. In addition, the epidemic has spawned an AIDS industry of consultants, not-for-profit organizations, and others (Figure 9).

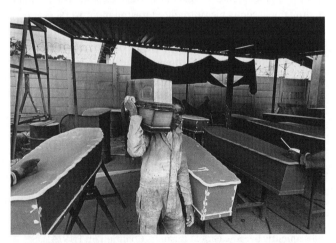

9. An unidentified man works in a coffin-making factory on May 2, 2003 in Soweto, South Africa. The country saw a big increase in funerals with about one thousand people are dying of HIV/AIDS every day. The role out of treatment has greatly reduced mortality.

Subsistence agriculture and the 'new variant famine' hypothesis

The majority of people in high-prevalence countries live in rural areas and are primarily dependent on subsistence agriculture. In Zambia and Zimbabwe, 64 per cent and 62 per cent, respectively, are rural dwellers. Exceptions are Botswana and South Africa where 61 per cent and 63 per cent are urban. In general rural populations are less well-served with health facilities, which means illness may be more common, last longer, and be more severe.

There is evidence AIDS is having an adverse effect on agriculture, mainly, but not only, through the impact on labour. Agricultural production, even most basic subsistence small holdings, does not operate in a vacuum. AIDS means key services such as marketing cooperatives and agricultural extension may be less efficient due to staff illness and death, and possibly declining morale. Illness among subsistence farmers means high-value and nutritious crops, such as cereals and oilseeds, are replaced by low-value and less nutritious ones that are easier to cultivate. The area planted may be reduced. There is an impact on animal husbandry: livestock get less attention.

Examples from Southern Africa show how AIDS has impacted agriculture. In Zambia's Central Province, the effect of adult illness and death on farm production was assessed among smallholder cotton farming households between 1999 and 2003. There were high levels of death and illness, 40 per cent of households had an adult death in the study period and 36 per cent reported an adult was sick 'regularly'. Where households experienced the death of a previously healthy, working-age adult the amount of land planted to maize declined by 16 per cent and that under cotton by 11 per cent. Across the border in a Zimbabwean communal farming area, a study found an adult

Production and people

death resulted in a 45 per cent decline in a household's marketed maize. Where the cause of death was identified as AIDS the loss was 61 per cent.

In Malawi prevalence in adults (aged 15 to 49) was 10 per cent in the early 2000s. A Care International survey in the Central Region found a significant number of households suffered from chronic illness. They were unable to provide the labour needed for even low productivity subsistence agriculture. Between 22 per cent and 64 per cent of households in study sites suffered from sickness, leading to loss of labour. In these households, 45 per cent delayed agricultural operations, 23 per cent left land fallow, and 26 per cent changed the crop mix. Resources were used for health care and funerals, and led to even lower levels of household income and nutrition. Female-headed households were worst affected as women do much of the agricultural work and combine this with childbearing and rearing, and household responsibilities. They have the 'double burden of care': they are most likely to suffer from HIV and AIDS, and they are responsible for caring for others.

The picture that emerges from Malawi is of an increasingly malnourished, stressed society. There is long-term environmental degradation: 85 per cent of energy comes from traditional fuel, mainly wood, leading to massive deforestation. Fish production from Lake Malawi has declined from about 30,000 tons a year in the late 20th century to just about 2,000 tons a year currently, which is particularly significant since fish contributed 70 per cent of the total animal protein consumption. There are frequent and severe climatic events. The drought of 2001 to 2003 led Alex de Waal and I to postulate in a *Lancet* article that the AIDS epidemic had such far-reaching adverse implications and interactions with the drought that it could lead to 'new variant famine'. In a 2015 article 'The 2001–03 Famine and the Dynamics of HIV in Malawi: A Natural Experiment', Michael Loevinsohn looks at the effect of that famine. He concluded the Malawi famine had a rapid and substantial effect on HIV prevalence, mainly through migration and increased transactional sex.

The country recovered but in 2015 southern Malawi was devastated by the worst floods in living memory, which affected more than a million people: 336,000 who were displaced; 100 people killed; and an estimated 64,000 hectares of cropland were washed away. In 2016 the country faced another severe drought.

When the first edition of this VSI was produced in 2008, I speculated that Malawi might provide an example of AIDS as a cause of state failure. This has not been the case, the resilience of societies is remarkable. Writing of AIDS and agricultural output, Seeley looks at Uganda and notes:

> HIV needs to be seen in the context of everyday life and the many challenges posed by poverty, crop disease, weather conditions and accidents and illness...HIV does not stand apart from other forms of sickness and misfortune; the ways in which people manage and continue to cope with the effects of the epidemic draw upon their experience of managing other problems and other forms of uncertainty. Placing HIV against this broader canvas enables us to appreciate the many challenges people face and to understand that the impact of the epidemic cannot be viewed in isolation from these events.

Across the world the pressure caused by AIDS needs to be seen in the context of other stressors. The most important one for subsistence farmers is climate change. As with AIDS, vulnerability to climate change is differentiated and it is the poor who are most exposed. In Africa the manifestation of climate change is less reliable, shorter, and later rains. The consequence is that the window of opportunity to plough and plant is decreased, and if someone is sick at the crucial time then this can be catastrophic as no crops will be harvested for a year.

Malnutrition has adverse implications in high HIV prevalence settings. Nutritional status is a determinant of risk of transmission both between adults and from mothers to infants. Undernourished people are more likely to be infected. Those who are infected endanger their health by going hungry. HIV replicates more rapidly in malnourished individuals, hastening the progression from HIV to AIDS. People living with HIV have greater nutritional requirements, needing more protein and energy. There is a vicious cycle, some illnesses reduce appetite and even ability to eat—oral candidiasis being an example—and others such as diarrhoea inhibit the absorption of nutrients. A further complication is it has become apparent, with the roll out of treatment, that in order for people to adhere and get the maximum benefit from the drugs they need food. Taking ART on an empty stomach leads to nausea and makes the drugs less effective.

The issue is not simply overall availability of food, but also the ability of the poorest members of society to purchase it. This is especially the case in urban areas. Zimbabwe provides an extreme example. The Famine Early Warning Systems Network warned, in March 2006, that macro-economic collapse had put the cost of basic foodstuffs beyond the reach of most Zimbabweans. The drought returned in 2014/15 when farmers produced 742,226 tonnes of maize as against 1,456,153 tonnes the previous season. In mid-2015 the government needed at least US$300 million to import enough grain to avert hunger. The 2015/16 rains failed across Southern Africa.

Families and households

The first consequence of an infection is stress. No matter who is HIV+ the question is: how did they come to be infected? Stories across the world tell of the devastation an HIV diagnosis can bring. HIV is often identified through antenatal testing or when an infant is sickly. Thus the infection is gendered—because women are first to be diagnosed they are assumed to have brought it into the family. At worst it can lead to bitter family break-up. Those who argue for massive voluntary testing campaigns should not underestimate the stigma and shame associated with what is a deadly, sexually transmitted infection.

Illness initially affects individuals. Sick adults can't engage in productive work. This includes paid and unpaid employment as well as housework and child care. It means people are less able to engage in community activities, the warp and weft of social reproduction. But it is not just the labour that is lost, the sick need care. Some help may be provided through state social and medical services. Where this is not available, care has to come from the family and community (most usually the family). This means that spouses care for each other, children care for their parents, and the elderly tend their children and grandchildren. Most care is provided by women and is generally not recognized as 'real' work. The idea that families will provide care is hardly revolutionary, it happens out of necessity all the time. AIDS, however, is costly, and can have a bleak prognosis. This disease is causing huge trauma across households and communities.

The inability of an adult to work means less income or production. The initial response is to change resource use. If the family has been saving that will stop. Expenditures are reduced. People eat fewer meals, with a lower range and quality of food. Possessions may be sold, or the family may borrow. If the household is forced to sell the assets used in production (ploughs, oxen, or a sewing machine) chances of recovery are reduced.

Shocks to households are not unusual, and much has been written on this topic. People face droughts, earthquakes, floods, tsunamis, illness, and other catastrophes. There are coping mechanisms that come into play. Unsurprisingly, the better resourced a household is at the outset, the better it will be able to cope. AIDS is different because of the long periods of illness.

As the pandemic progressed, especially prior to treatment, the burden increasingly fell on the older women, particularly maternal grandparents. Sick people returned home with their children, to be cared for by parents. Work in Warwick Junction in Durban by Chazan found older women were unevenly and increasingly burdened by AIDS, bearing the brunt of the social, care-taking, economic, and emotional burdens of their families. Two-thirds of those interviewed had cared for family members or neighbours sick with AIDS. The older women in this study suffered from (largely untreated) chronic illnesses such as diabetes, arthritis, and hypertension, and feared personal illness, not just for themselves, but because of what it would mean for their families.

The myth of coping

An HIV diagnosis has huge implications for any individual, but in general it is at the household level that the worst impacts of AIDS are visible. One of the main factors which exacerbate the impoverishment of people is the burden of care. Most affected households do not, in an identifiable sense, 'cope', but rather they 'struggle', and they do this because they have no other choice. In addition, households, especially rural ones, are obliged to carry the burden that is 'shifted' from the formal sector and urban areas. The unstated assumption is that 'wider society' will carry the burden. 'Wider society' in this context is chiefly women in rural areas and urban slums. ART can change this picture. If people can access drugs and adhere to them then the illness and deaths that were so overwhelming fifteen years ago can be averted. However for the patients even where the drugs are free, and currently they are generally provided by governments or international agencies, there are additional costs: transport, nutritious food, and lost days of work.

Chapter 6
Development, numbers, and politics

Development and targets

Development is about more than macro-economic growth. This was well articulated in the UNDP's first 'Human Development Report' (HDR) in 1990, which stated: 'The real wealth of a nation is its people. And the purpose of development is to create an enabling environment for people to enjoy long, healthy and creative lives.' The report introduced the Human Development Index (HDI), a composite number constructed from three indices: life expectancy, educational attainment, and standard of living. This has evolved. (Box 4.)

The first HDR noted: 'The AIDS epidemic poses a serious threat to all countries, but it particularly affects developing countries that lack preventive health and social support services and that have a high incidence of infection. It adds burdens to debt, poverty, illiteracy, structural adjustment and other diseases'. The effect of AIDS on the HDI was not considered until 1997. When it was factored in rankings and scores changed immediately and significantly. Botswana dropped from 71st rank in 1997 to 131st in 2003. Its HDI went from 0.681 in 1990 to 0.565 in 2003. Data were subsequently 'retrofitted' in UNDP publications, and in these Botswana's HDI falls steadily between 1990 and 2000 (instead of the precipitous drop described previously).

Box 4 The HDI and MDGs

The HDI is a summary measure of average achievement in key dimensions of human development: a long and healthy life, being knowledgeable, and having a decent standard of living. Its calculation, which has over time become more sophisticated, is based on:

- The health dimension which is assessed by life expectancy at birth. This component of the HDI is calculated using a minimum value of 20 years and maximum value of 85 years.
- The education component of the HDI is measured by mean of years of schooling for adults aged 25 years and expected years of schooling for children of school entering age.
- The standard of living dimension is measured by gross national income per capita.

The UNDP notes the failings and limitations of each of these measures.

The eight MDGs were the first international development targets. They were set by the United Nations in 2000, to run to 2015. These goals were intended to be realistic and achievable and were:

1. Eradicating extreme poverty and hunger
2. Achieving universal primary education
3. Promoting gender equality and empowering women
4. Reducing child mortality
5. Improving maternal health
6. Combating HIV/AIDS, malaria, and other diseases
7. Ensuring environmental sustainability
8. Develop a global partnership for development

Goal 6 was most relevant to this book. Goals 4 and 5 were directly related to health. Goal 3 had obvious implications for AIDS responses especially with regard to prevention. More

When the MDGs were set it was not fully appreciated that AIDS
would make achieving some of them difficult, specifically in high
HIV prevalence countries. The child mortality target, reducing
under-5 deaths by two-thirds between 1990 and 2015, was
worst affected. In Lesotho, an extreme case, this fell to 88.1 per
1,000 in 1990, then rose to 123.4 in 2005 before falling to
93.6 in 2013—still higher than twenty-three years before. Goal 6
was specifically to combat the three diseases AIDS, malaria,
and TB. However they remain the primary cause of premature
death in some countries.

In the third decade of the epidemic there is still little appreciation
of what HIV and AIDS meant and means for development targets.
There are reasons: indicators are based on historical data and
don't take account of future impact; the data do not compare
'with' and 'without AIDS' scenarios; there are a limited number
of countries where impact has been significant; and most
importantly, advent of treatment means morbidity and mortality
are reduced, but costs (which are usually not borne by patients
or, in some cases, even governments) are not visible.

The Millennium Development Goal (MDG) era passed. In
September 2015 the nations of the world adopted the Sustainable
Development Goals (SDGs) to replace the MDGs. There are
seventeen goals broken down into 169 specific targets. Their
overarching aim is to wipe out extreme poverty and hunger by
2030, and to protect the planet from degradation and
environmental catastrophe (five of the goals relate to climate
change). (Box 5.)

Box 5 The health SDG

There is only one specific health goal (number 3): to ensure healthy lives and promote well-being for all at all ages. The targets related to HIV and AIDS are: reduce the global maternal mortality ratio to less than 70 per 100,000 live births; end preventable deaths of newborns and children under 5; reduce neonatal mortality to 12 per 1,000 live births and under-5 mortality to 25 per 1,000 live births; end the epidemics of AIDS, TB, malaria, and neglected tropical diseases and combat hepatitis, water-borne, and other communicable diseases; strengthen the prevention and treatment of substance abuse; ensure universal access to sexual and reproductive health care services, achieve universal health coverage; support research and development of, and provide access to, vaccines and medicines; increase health financing and recruitment, development, training, and retention of the health workforce in developing countries; and strengthen the capacity for early warning, risk reduction, and management of health risks.

There have been critiques of the SDG agenda including accusations that they are watered down MDGs, will perpetuate status quo, and that the price tag, US$3 trillion, is unachievable. Some feel there are too many SDGs and far too many targets. It is certain though, with the emphasis on reducing poverty and addressing environmental threats, that health in general and HIV specifically have moved down the global agenda, in stark contrast to the prominence the disease had over the first fifteen years of the millennium.

The golden age of specific AIDS goals

In January 2000, for the first time, a disease (AIDS) was discussed in a special session of the UN Security Council. US Vice President Al Gore said: 'it [HIV] threatens not just individual citizens, but the very institutions that define and defend the character of a society. This disease weakens workforces and saps economic strength. AIDS strikes at teachers, and denies education to their students. It strikes at the military, and subverts the forces of order and peacekeeping.' Six months later the Security Council passed Resolution 1308, recognizing that the spread of HIV and AIDS could have a 'uniquely devastating impact' on all sectors and levels of society, and pose a risk to stability and security.

Two months before the resolution the UN General Assembly Special Session (UNGASS) on HIV/AIDS, UN Secretary-General Kofi Annan had called for the creation of a 'global war chest' to finance MDG 6. UNGASS resulted in the first UN Political Declaration on HIV/AIDS and committed to the establishment of a global HIV and health fund. Crucially, civil society was among the stakeholders who charted how the AIDS component of MDG 6 would be achieved. Prevention was the mainstay of the response. In January 2002 the Global Fund to Fight AIDS, Tuberculosis and Malaria opened for business in Geneva with the clarion cry of 'Raise it, spend it, prove it'.

Money flowed. In 2003 Republican President George W. Bush pledged US$15 billion toward the Presidential Emergency Program for AIDS Relief (PEPFAR). Writing in 2015, Bush provides an explanation for this extraordinary intervention. He said, 'As President I found it morally unacceptable for the United States to stand aside while millions of people died from a disease we could treat. I also recognized that saving lives in Africa serves America's strategic interests. When societies abroad are healthier and more prosperous they are more stable and secure.'

Later that year, on World AIDS Day (1 December), WHO and UNAIDS launched the '3 × 5' campaign to provide antiretroviral treatment to three million people in developing and transition countries by the end of 2005. Although the target was not achieved, the ground work for expanding treatment, both practical and political, was done.

In the 2006 Political Declaration on HIV/AIDS, the UN pledged to work for universal access to HIV prevention, treatment, care, and support, and affordable ART. Two years later the UN High-Level Meeting on AIDS recognized the importance of populations at higher risk: sex workers, MSM, transgender people, and IDUs. In 2011 the theme was developing targets to run concurrently with those of MDG 6 and the pledge to reduce sexual HIV transmission and transmission among IDUs by 50 per cent; eliminate new infections among children; place fifteen million people on ART; and halve TB deaths among people living with HIV—all by 2015.

The UNAIDS 'Fast Track: Ending the AIDS Epidemic by 2030' paper set targets for 2020 and 2030. These are that, by 2020, 90 per cent of HIV-infected people should know their status; 90 per cent of these be receiving treatment; and 90 per cent of those on treatment have a suppressed viral load. This means that there would be 500,000 new infections in 2020 with 27 per cent of these infected people having unsuppressed viral loads. Ending the epidemic by 2030 would mean 95 per cent knowing their status; 95 per cent being on treatment; and 95 per cent being virally suppressed. This would mean virtually no vertical infections, but still 200,000 new infections among adults (as compared to 2.1 million in 2013). UNAIDS believes this could avert twenty-eight million infections and twenty-one million deaths up to 2030, and save US\$24 billion which would otherwise be needed for HIV treatment. A rapid scale-up in interventions up to 2020 is crucial in this approach, with more money and effort needed over the five years to 2020—a significant political commitment.

Politics

HIV and AIDS mix sex, death, fear, and disease in ways that can be interpreted to suit different prejudices and agendas. AIDS was (and still is) used to stigmatize groups. Health responses to epidemic outbreaks focus on technical and scientific answers. The popular images are of squads of epidemiologists arriving to locate the source of disease, and medical task teams following to treat patients. This biomedical attitude to infectious disease was reinforced by the Ebola outbreak. We want to believe there are quick technical, scientific solutions to epidemics—because, if there are, then we can buy them, use them, and move on.

AIDS has become an endemic and well-understood disease. However the politics of the epidemic are complex and continue to feed into the response. We need to understand the underlying causes, as discussed in Chapter 3. Providing good health is messy, intricate, and about sustainable development, equity, and justice. It needs political engagement—decisions about treatment and prevention, and who gets what.

AIDS, conflict, and security

One early advocacy platform was to present the concept of HIV/AIDS as representing a security risk, which was put forward in the early 1990s. I was one of those who made this argument. We postulated AIDS was linked with conflict because armed forces (regular armies, militias, and rebels) had high HIV prevalence, and were more likely to engage in risky sexual behaviours and rape. We predicted economic slowdown and substantial loss of skilled people and leadership. AIDS, we argued, had to have security implications. This became a rallying cry. In 1999 American Ambassador to the UN Richard Holbrooke visited Lusaka and was confronted by AIDS orphaning. This epiphany is believed to have influenced the January 2000 Security Council statement by Vice President Gore.

Intuitively it seemed situations of conflict would facilitate HIV spread, but as Pulitzer Prize-winning science writer Laurie Garrett pointed out, the idea does not stand up to scrutiny. In a time of conflict there may be less spread of communicable disease: trade decreases; borders close; and mobility, apart from that of refugees and armies, is diminished. It is peace, with renewed movement of people and reconstruction, that poses a bigger risk. A 2015 publication modelled the association between violent conflict and HIV incidence in thirty-six sub-Saharan Africa countries between 1990 and 2012. This found the HIV incidence rate had increased in the five years prior to conflict but that there was no evidence of an increase during and following violent conflict.

Analysts, including senior army officers, suggested in the early years of the epidemic that HIV/AIDS might undermine military effectiveness. In 2006, with colleagues Alex de Waal and Tsadkan Gebre-Tensae, I revisited this and published an assessment of the risks of infection in militaries. Again, one of the accepted shibboleths was that military populations had a high prevalence of HIV. We concluded that this was not the case. Armed forces are primarily made up of young men who have low levels of infection. Most militaries test recruits (although few admit it), some may test repeatedly. Being HIV+ usually excludes a person from recruitment and may result in service being terminated. Armed forces can educate, control, and even 'grow' an infection-free workforce.

Most assessments of AIDS and security consisted largely of a catalogue of reasons why the epidemic *might* lead to crises. Such warnings were appropriate in the 1990s, when there were little data and much speculation. Academics Tony Barnett and Gwyn Prins of the London School of Economics pointed to the use of 'factoids'—frequently reported statements which then are deemed to be truth—in their UNAIDS report 'HIV/AIDS and Security: Fact, Fiction & Evidence'. Of greater concern is the impact of conflict and political instability on prevention and treatment.

The numbers game

The early history of HIV was driven by media hype. How many cases were there? Where were they? Who was being infected and why? The first cases in the West were identified in groups of people that shared behaviours (gay men and drug users); specific nationalities (Haitians in the US); and those who received contaminated blood products. As the ways in which HIV was transmitted were understood, the focus shifted from identifiable categories of people to identifiable behaviours.

Initially the data were highly political. No country wanted to be identified with the epidemic. The most blatant example of cooking the figures was in the late 1980s. Zimbabwe officially notified the WHO that they had several hundred cases of AIDS. Shortly afterwards South Africa reported 120 cases. Within days Zimbabwe revised its figure to 119, not wanting to exceed the number reported by the racist regime to the south. Another response was simply to deny the figures. India did this by refusing to allow UNAIDS to publish an estimate of total infections in the 2004 global report. The 2015 UNAIDS data give only upper and lower estimates of people living with HIV for Russia.

Do data matter? They do if debates about figures prevent action and advocacy or provide an excuse for delay. Numbers really matter for funders if they are to continue to offer support. PEPFAR committed, between 2004 and 2015, a staggering US$65,921 million, with a 2016 request for US$6,542 million. They have to show results, and indeed PEPFAR data show, in 2014, they were supporting 7.7 million people on ART (4.5 million were receiving direct support and 3.2 million benefited from technical support). Their backing provided HIV testing and counselling for more than 14.2 million pregnant women, and treatment for the 749,313 women who tested positive. They funded more than 6.5 million medical male circumcisions in Eastern and Southern Africa.

At the global level we need to track progress towards the target of ending AIDS. What are the numbers? Where are they? Who is paying and how much is it costing? Decisions as to where to put resources are dependent on more than data—they are political and economic—but accurate numbers are important, as is being increasingly recognized by the GF and UNAIDS.

The political impact

It is clear that potential political impact is limited. The best data come from the Democracy in Africa Research Unit (DARU) at the University of Cape Town. DARU collaborates with the University of Michigan on the Afro-barometer project measuring the social, political, and economic atmosphere in Africa through national public attitude surveys.

Political fallout could be through loss of leaders and voters, changing voting patterns, and disengagement and disillusionment with the political process, at all levels from national to municipal. In the early years there was evidence of increased mortality among politicians. In Zambia between 1964 and 1984 there were fourteen by-elections caused by deaths of parliamentarians, between 1984 and 2003 there were fifty-nine deaths, thirty-nine between 1993 and 2003, when AIDS mortality was increasing. ART changed this, and it is not surprising that politicians are among the first to access treatment.

According to the Afro-barometer surveys, HIV and AIDS are not important as political or election issues. Indeed people's primary problems are unemployment and poverty. In the first round of surveys AIDS featured on the public agenda of only three Southern African countries: 24 per cent of Batswana, 14 per cent of Namibians, and 13 per cent of South Africans cited HIV/AIDS as one of the top three problems facing the country. The question posed subsequently was: 'In your opinion, what are the most important problems facing this country that government should address?' Only in Botswana was AIDS seen as a significant issue, but by round six which began in 2014, only 1.1 per cent of Batswana mentioned it. In all countries, except Lesotho, more than half the citizens think governments are doing well in combatting AIDS, in the case of Botswana 95 per cent are satisfied with the government's response.

One clear early result of the epidemic was activism. This began in the gay community in the US. Horrified by the illnesses and deaths among friends, they mobilized and in 1987 formed the AIDS Coalition to Unleash Power (ACT-UP) highlighting high drug prices and inadequate responses. This activism was mirrored in the UK—the Terrence Higgins Trust was formed in 1982 to personalize and humanize AIDS.

In the resource-poor world the Treatment Action Campaign (TAC) was launched in South Africa in 1998. In 2002, it was able to take the ANC government to court and win over government policies on access to medicines for pregnant women. In Uganda the AIDS Support Organization (TASO), established in 1987, grew into one of the major care-providing organizations. In Brazil activists brought prices of drugs down. One of *the* defining features of AIDS was the strengthening of civil society and grass roots responses. This led to the development of numerous NGOs and social movements. These range from orphan support to home-based care groups, to lobbying and advocacy movements pressing for reduced drug prices.

However, AIDS does not unite people politically—there is no HIV party! It does not lead to collapse nor to dramatic change. While the direct links between AIDS and politics may be hard to identify and measure there are possible indirect ones. Social scientists identify three key factors for sustaining and consolidating democratic rule. It is harder for poor countries to maintain democracy. Contracting economies and growing inequality threaten democratic processes. Second, there need to be strong political institutions including civil services, judiciaries, and executives. Third are the attitudes: people must want democracy. AIDS could affect all these factors.

A 2014 book by Šehović on sovereignty, responsibility, and AIDS, argues that the state has an obligation for 'awarding and enacting' the rights of its constituents (including health); is the ultimate guarantor of these rights; and where the state cannot do this the international community has to intervene or assume some responsibility. However, the question of how to claim these rights remains vexing.

Natural and human disasters

The real political impact may come from ensuring treatment is available and affordable. There is ample evidence of the importance of adherence to reduce viral load and improve clinical prognosis. Increased risk of illness and death among those who are poorly adherent were shown in South Africa. Patients obtaining less than 80 per cent of their prescription refills were over three times more likely to die than those getting more than 80 per cent.

The evidence suggests patients in resource-poor settings are as adherent as those in the wealthy world, provided drugs are available. However, unfavourable contexts limit an individual's control over their own treatment. In particular, inconsistent drug supplies are an important factor. Here, the public health, social, and economic environment is critical.

The goal of ensuring people remain adherent assumes that drugs are available. There are different crises that can potentially undermine access, including government inefficiencies and corruption. Writing with colleagues in 2013, I addressed how to reconcile the science and policy divide in scaling up ART. We looked at South Africa, which while it has the highest burden of HIV, also has one of the best health care systems in Africa. We identified the issues as being governance, human resources for health, and infrastructural and fiscal constraints.

In South Africa the three spheres of governance are: national, provincial, and local. Delivery is at provincial or local level but policy is set at the national level causing disconnects. Human resources for health are generally constrained: the majority of the doctors seek to practice in urban centres. Of course the picture for the continent is darker. Liberia has two doctors per 100,000 people; the US has 245 for the same number. Infrastructural constraints include where facilities are located and how they operate. Our conclusion was that although South Africa had the largest ART delivery programme in the world, it was creaking and further expansion would require attention to unresolved issues.

In 2010, I and others assessed unexpected situations that might compromise ART adherence in Southern and Eastern Africa—although this has wider application. These are of different natures, durations (short-term vs long-term), and geographical extent (localized vs widespread). We looked at problems with health system functioning and ART delivery during the 2008 floods in Mozambique; the public sector strike in South Africa; and the political and economic crisis in Zimbabwe.

In natural disasters, health concerns are dominated by sanitary problems and overcrowding in camps. There is increased risk of diarrhoeal diseases, cholera, measles, and malaria. The immediate need is for safe access to clean water and food, which means other health problems are eclipsed. Displacement means those on ART may not be able to access their medication. In Mozambique, following the 2008 floods, Médecins Sans Frontières (MSF) reported that sixty patients in Mutarara (Tete province) on HIV and TB treatment were missing and had not come to collect their monthly medication. Teams were sent out to find the patients. Most public health services do not have the capacity to respond in this way.

The category of health system or service failure manifests in many ways. Common examples include health worker strikes and drug stock-outs. South Africa has one of the better public health systems in Africa but a month-long public sector strike in 2007 meant patients could not get drugs. The fragility of the health system was further illustrated in December 2012 when, owing to severe drug supply and delivery disruptions, MSF had to step in to supply the Mthatha (Eastern Cape) medical depot with ART for 50,000 patients. An estimated 5,494 adults went at least one day without treatment.

Political and economic failure has widespread implications for the health system and is harder to manage. Health care provision becomes more difficult due to the lack of drugs, medical supplies, and insufficient health workers. In Zimbabwe, in 2008, this resulted in the closure of some of the largest hospitals. In conflicts, routine health delivery is one of the services affected. Not only is it more difficult for medical staff to function, as their personal safely may be at risk, but there is greater demand for emergency services, and supply chains are disrupted. Patients may not be able to access facilities and ART may not be a priority.

Good national and international programmes need to take these issues into account. No one wants to face the disruptions described previously, but they will occur and it is best to be prepared, especially when the consequences of non-adherence are so severe both for the patients and the health system more broadly. One of the greatest dangers is the development of a drug-resistant HIV, which may then be transmitted. The solutions include proper supply chain management. Keeping buffer stocks is a good strategy, which in an ideal world could be done regionally. Bringing treatment closer to the patients and enabling nurses to prescribe or provide ART will facilitate access.

Chapter 7
Treatment and prevention dilemmas

The public health context

The best way to achieve a healthy society is to ensure people don't fall ill or have accidents. Successful prevention and public health programmes are the paramount and the most cost effective way to health. Persuading people to never smoke means rates of lung cancer will plummet; wearing seatbelts reduces the risk of injury in motor accidents. There will, of course, still be disease, natural disaster, and accidents, when medical interventions remain essential.

The role of public health is to keep people healthy at a population level. In a seminal 2014 *Lancet* article, Davies and colleagues identify four historical waves of public health development and suggested a new wave is in the making. Each wave overlaps and builds on previous gains. The ideas have global application and are particularly pertinent to HIV.

The first wave (1830 to 1900) was structural. Physical and environmental conditions were addressed, including provision of clean water, sewerage disposal, food safety, and improved working conditions. The often cited example is of physician John Snow identifying a pump in Broad Street in Soho, London, as the primary source of a cholera outbreak in 1854. Once the handle was removed the number of cases fell rapidly.

The second wave (1890 to 1950) was biomedical and scientific advance. Its crucial foundation was the first vaccine (smallpox) administered in 1796, and the UK's 1853 Vaccination Act which made immunization compulsory for infants by the age of 3 months. In the 20th century, vaccines against diphtheria, measles, mumps, rubella, and polio were developed. Vaccination is still a major contributor in lowering morbidity and mortality, especially among children, across the world.

The third wave of advance (1940 to 1980) was clinical. Growing understanding of causes of disease resulted in lifestyle interventions, two examples being the relationship between smoking and cancer, and diet and diabetes.

The fourth wave began in 1960, with examination of the social determinants of health, and understanding that ill health generally has roots in economic and social factors. This was endorsed by the WHO's 2008 Commission report, 'Closing the Gap in a Generation: Health Equity through Action on the Social Determinants of Health'.

The fifth wave of public health development, the authors argue, should be 'a culture for health'. Health should be the norm; valued and incentivized; healthy choices the default; and unhealthy activities actively discouraged. This requires involvement of individuals, the community, government at every level—institutions and the private sector, all actively nudging people towards well-being.

In the AIDS world there has been a vigorous debate over the role of treatment in prevention and where resources should be concentrated. This is made more complex by cost of treatment and relative poverty of those countries where the burden of disease is highest. The 2015 UNAIDS-*Lancet* Commission on 'Defeating AIDS—Advancing Global Health' argued that the epidemic is still a major threat to public health: 'Too many people are becoming newly infected with HIV, too many people do not know that they have HIV and too many people are dying from AIDS-related causes.... With still more new HIV infections each year than patients who start ART [antiretroviral therapies], the AIDS response appears to be running at a standstill.'

The founding director of UNAIDS, Peter Piot, wrote in 2015: 'As with most health and social issues, prevention has often been neglected in favour of treatment. Yet we will not treat ourselves out of this epidemic. HIV prevention must be reinvigorated, particularly for people at highest risk of infection, while ensuring the legal and societal discrimination of these populations is removed'.

The concept of an 'AIDS transition', developed by Mead Over of the Centre of Global Development in Washington, is blindingly simple. Figure 10 shows that, until the number of new infections falls below the number of deaths of HIV infected people, from whatever cause, the numbers needing treatment will rise (the gap between the lines). If the two lines do not cross, the number will

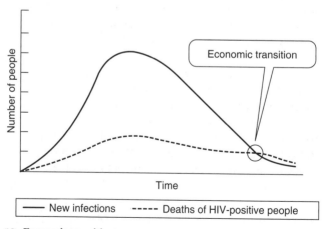

10. **Economic transition.**

continue to grow. This is a nightmare for both health and finance ministries. When the transition is achieved, the ministries can plan ahead with certainty.

HIV prevention

HIV infection is preventable. The period from 2001 to 2013 saw the number of new infections decline by 38 per cent to 2.1 million, and the trend continues. UNAIDS seeks to end AIDS by 2030. The first biomedical strategy was to ensure safe blood and blood products by screening donors and testing donations. Blood safety is generally not an issue except in emergency situations.

The first social interventions concerned behaviour change, advising people to use condoms, have fewer partners, and practice monogamy or abstinence. This applied to heterosexual couples and MSMs. In the UK, Health Secretary Norman Fowler, who served through the early years of the epidemic from 1981 to 1987, led a remarkably effective campaign—against the wishes of Prime Minister Margret Thatcher and those of the cabinet who wanted a moral line drawn against promiscuity, infidelity, and 'sexual deviation' (i.e. homosexuality). Under Fowler, a leaflet with the strapline 'Don't die of ignorance' was delivered to every household. This was bold and effective. (Figure 11.)

Other early evidence of interventional success came from Thailand. Here the '100% condom programme' required compulsory, consistent condom use in brothels. Indicators were that condom use in brothels increased to over 90 per cent by 1992, and cases of male STIs at government clinics decreased from 200,000 in 1989 to 20,000 in 1995. HIV prevalence among pregnant women peaked at 2.35 per cent in 1995, and was just 0.5 per cent in 2014.

Condoms are a biomedical intervention, but ensuring an adequate supply requires planning, and then persuading people to use

11. AIDS poster.

them consistently and correctly needs behaviour change. Male condoms reduce heterosexual transmission by at least 80 per cent and offer 64 per cent protection in anal sex among MSMs. There are few data for female condoms but they are believed to have a similar impact.

In the case of IDUs, provision of clean needles, sterilization equipment, and discouraging needle sharing is effective. Longer term opioid substitution therapy with methadone or buprenorphine is an effective form of treatment for opioid dependence. Unfortunately the criminalization of drugs and the stigma around their use has meant that only a few far-sighted authorities took a pragmatic public health approach. They included Scotland and Australia.

Crucial to behaviour change is community mobilization and leadership. Such proactive ownership of risk management was seen early in the epidemic in the gay community. This is true of all prevention methods including treatment, in every setting, as will be discussed. It is an important and neglected issue.

Prevention of vertical transmission began in 1994. There has been exceptional progress recently. The proportion of pregnant women living with HIV who receive ART medicines doubled over the five years from 2009 to 2014, from 33 per cent to 68 per cent. Drugs and treatment regimens continue to advance.

Medical male circumcision reduces the chance of HIV infection for uninfected men by up to 66 per cent: it is a one-off intervention and gives lifelong protection. As fewer men are infected, the risks for women will be reduced. Both condoms and circumcision are largely male controlled although mothers could be encouraged to have male infants circumcised.

The need for female-controlled HIV prevention led to the development of a microbicide. While, as discussed earlier, these have been shown to work in some trials, in real-world settings women do not seem to be adherent. The challenge seems to be to facilitate women in using the gels consistently.

As discussed in Chapter 2, in 2011, Treatment as Prevention (TasP) was announced as a 'game changer'. ART reduces the HIV viral load in the blood, semen, vaginal fluid, and rectal fluid to very low or even undetectable levels, thus reducing an individual's risk of HIV transmission. Prevention can become targeted towards behaviours that make people vulnerable to infection—the 'key populations', who need special attention. Globally MSMs are nineteen times, injecting drug users twenty-eight times, and sex workers twelve times more likely to be infected than the general population. The 1987 British leaflet campaign was appropriate on the basis of available evidence. Today it would be a waste of resources.

One recent innovation is mapping geographic infection hot spots. The Africa Centre for Health and Population Studies located in Matubatuba in Northern KwaZulu-Natal, South Africa, led the way. Unsurprisingly, they show areas sending or receiving migrants, and settlements proximate to major roads have the highest incidence rates. The most recent data reported by

UNAIDS in their 2015 World AIDS Day report, 'Focus on Location and Population', show that living in a community on KwaZulu-Natal with 30 to 40 per cent ART coverage reduced a person's HIV risk by 38 per cent, compared with living in an area with under 10 per cent ART coverage. Each single percentage point increase in ART coverage reduced HIV risk by 1.45 per cent.

The identification of particular at-risk groups and locations means prevention campaigns can be targeted, effective, and cost-effective. In generalized epidemics, the target population, numbers, and areas will be significantly larger than the concentrated epidemics embedded in localized risk groups. Achieving control of the epidemic means: doing the right thing, in the right place, at the right time, to the right target.

Ultimately, the structural factors that drive an epidemic need to be addressed. The British Department for International Development grasped this in funding the STRIVE Research Consortium which investigates the social norms and inequalities that drive HIV. The upstream structural determinants being researched include: gender inequality and violence; poor livelihood options; alcohol availability and drinking norms; and stigma and criminalization. Understanding these factors is not enough. What is needed is to appropriately address the complex issues; to communicate and persuade effectively; and, especially, to establish how interventions can be taken to scale in a cost-effective manner.

AIDS treatment development

Once HIV was identified, work began on finding treatments. AZT was approved 1987, taking only twenty-five months from discovery to approval, and found to be effective in preventing HIV transmission from mother to child and after needle stick injuries. Unfortunately the virus quickly mutated and developed resistance to AZT.

In 1996, the breakthrough of using three drugs in combination was announced. This dramatically reduced morbidity and mortality in rich countries. The drugs were, however, very expensive, at US$10,000 per patient per year. The result was they were beyond the reach of people in the resource-poor world. This was due largely to the stranglehold monopoly of major pharmaceutical companies and patents that prevented low-cost manufacturers from entering the market.

The theme for the 2000 IAC in Durban was, 'Breaking the Silence', a call to talk about and act on equal access to treatment and care and improved prevention. There was increasing activism and outrage about the prices of drugs. In 2001, the Doha declaration on the Trade Related Aspects of Intellectual Property Rights (TRIPS) Agreement and Public Health was adopted by World Trade Organisation member states. This created a mechanism for WTO members to issue compulsory licences in order to export generic versions of patented medicines to countries without manufacturing capacity. Just prior to this, the Indian manufacturer of generic drugs, Cipla, announced they would sell triple therapy for US$350 per person per year. With increasing numbers of pharmaceutical companies, primarily from India, entering the market, the price of drugs continued to fall and treatment regimens became simpler: three active ingredients combined in a daily tablet. Indeed, a once a week pill or implant should be available soon.

The drugs have side effects; some are minor, such as nausea, diarrhoea, and headaches, and disappear soon after treatment is initiated. Others are more serious and can worsen over time. These include nerve damage (peripheral neuropathy), liver and kidney damage (nephrotoxicity and hepatotoxicity), risk of cardiovascular events, and fat redistribution (lipodystrophy). If patients are not adherent then the virus will rapidly develop resistance, the viral load will climb, and they will fall ill. Being adherent requires taking at least 80 per cent of the drugs as prescribed when the regime is based on protease inhibitors and 95 per cent in the case of non-nucleoside-based therapies.

The previous discussion has focused on the amazing drugs developed with great speed in response to AIDS. However there is more to treatment than ART. Patients need to be identified as being HIV+, ideally through a blood test; they should be counselled on diagnosis and before starting treatment; their viral load and CD4 count needs to monitored. Once on drugs, provided they are doing well, this can be done as infrequently as once a year. In Malawi, MSF organized a 'viral load campaign' with the theme: 'know your viral load and be in control of your treatment'.

Co-infections, the most common of which is TB, may need treatment. Successful programmes encourage adherence and ensure patients are supported. This requires a health infrastructure and staff. The best way to ensure patients don't need second-line therapy is to make sure the first line works. The best way to prevent multidrug resistant TB is to treat all TB successfully.

Initially treatment was provided in 'vertical programmes' where the facilities focused on HIV. Increasingly, and as HIV is seen as a chronic condition, this is being done in 'horizontal programmes', via the standard public clinics. There are costs to this. In Durban, South Africa, the closure of McCord's Mission Hospital in 2013 meant that about 5,000 patients from the Sinikithemba HIV/AIDS Centre were transferred to the public sector. They commented on how much less personal attention they received. It is possible some of these patients ceased treatment and died.

The state of ART

There are two standards of treatment available. In the rich world, an HIV-infected person will have their virus strain identified, the appropriate mix and quantity of drugs prescribed, and their progress monitored to see how effective they are. This treatment is provided through national health services in most countries, by Medicaid or Medicare in the United States, or by the private sector. There are side effects but AIDS is treated as a long-term, chronic health condition by specialist HIV doctors. Indeed, as the cohort of infected people ages, the issue of HIV and the elderly is increasingly relevant.

In the resource-poor world, therapies are far more limited but treatment guidelines have evolved. When the '3 by 5' campaign was launched the target population were those patients with a CD4 count of less than 200. In 2010, evidence suggested treatment should be offered earlier, at a CD4 count of 350. The 2013 guidelines raised the level to 500. In 2015, the push was to put people on treatment as soon as they were identified as being HIV+. If patients develop resistance to first-line treatment, usually indicated by increased viral load, a second line can be given, costing double the first-line treatment. Should the patient develop resistance to the second line, where available, third-line or salvage therapy may be used, which costs fifteen times more.

The 'Vancouver Consensus' was written and released at the IAS's 8th International Conference on Pathogenesis, Treatment and Prevention in 2015. This stated:

> rather than waiting for immune deterioration, immediate antiretroviral (ARV) treatment more than doubles an individual's prospects of staying healthy and surviving. Offering ... antiretrovirals can prevent transmission from people living with HIV [and] ... protect[s] people at risk of infection through prophylactic use.
>
> Medical evidence is clear: All people living with HIV must have access to antiretroviral treatment upon diagnosis. Barriers [and] ... bias must be confronted and dismantled. And as part of a combination prevention effort, PrEP must be made available to protect those at high risk of acquiring HIV. The strategic use of

ARVs—through treatment and other preventive uses—can...move us vastly closer to our goal of ending the epidemic.

The ever earlier initiation of therapy has given rise to a new set of concerns: getting people on treatment, ensuring they are adherent, and monitoring drug resistance. A major issue in many settings is cost, even in the context of falling prices, as addressed in Chapter 8.

'How AIDS Changed Everything' noted that fifteen million people are receiving ART. However, 59 per cent of adults and 68 per cent of children who, under the guidelines, are eligible for treatment, are not accessing it. The first step is for people to know their HIV status. Women will be tested routinely if they receive antenatal care. One emerging issue has been babies protected at birth but who are subsequently infected in the first nine months. Preventing transmission to infants heralds the potential for an AIDS-free generation.

The treatment cascade is the number of people living with HIV who know their status, are receiving ART, and are virally suppressed. The evidence suggests that significant numbers of patients are lost at each stage. This illustrates the difficulties in encouraging and facilitating people in establishing their status, linking them to treatment, and ultimately supporting them in achieving suppressed viral loads. This is good for individual health and life opportunities, and effective in reducing transmission. Clearly, given the leakage at the various stages, there are challenges to using TasP at a population level.

The evidence suggests that people in poorer parts of the world are as likely to be adherent to treatment as those in wealthy countries. However taking treatment for the rest of one's life is hard. Seeley's work in East Africa notes the many barriers to accessing treatment. Getting to a clinic may involve transport costs and taking time off work or away from the fields for subsistence farmers. At many clinics, patients are required to wait for long periods, and a common complaint is that patients are treated disrespectfully by health staff. Getting and taking drugs may lead to stigma. One response is to travel to clinics further away in order to avoid being seen by friends and neighbours, which takes time and costs money. In some settings, people are reluctant to change behaviours if it draws attention to possible HIV infection: moderation of sexual activity and consumption of alcohol may imply the use of HIV drugs.

Seeley's work provides a longitudinal view of the epidemic, from ethnographic studies of households to demographic and health surveys. She notes:

> In three decades, the epidemic has moved from the management of death to the management of a chronic condition. This apparently smooth progression from ignorance to understanding belies the questions and insecurities that still operate at the individual level: will the medications work for me? If so will they continue to work? Will I suffer side-effects? Will I be susceptible to other illnesses? How will I cope with a lifelong condition?

Ways ahead

Prevention has to remain the priority. Although it is possible for HIV-infected people to live normal, productive lives, it is a personal challenge and it is expensive. This financial cost is an important issue in the resource-poor world: the drugs have to be taken for life and there is often stigma (including self-stigma) attached to being on the treatment.

It makes more sense to prevent a condition from occurring than to have to treat it. Some prevention activities have become routine: this includes blood and blood product safety, and prevention of vertical transmission. Other measures seem blindingly obvious, but politics and religion may play an unhelpful role. Examples of this are the reluctance to fund clean needles for IV drug use or methadone substitution in Russia; and homophobia and anti-gay legislation in a number of African countries and Russia, which have forced this at-risk group underground.

Providing treatment is an effective prevention tool. Treatment has changed the discourse around the epidemic and has given rise to new and important questions. These include: how government organizes prevention and treatment delivery; the role of profit-led pharmaceutical companies; who gets what treatment; who pays and for how long; what are the rights and responsibilities of infected people and the states they live in; the attitude of the international community; and are people with HIV being privileged over those with other conditions? Science has taken giant leaps. The question remains of how economic and political conditions will play out in the years ahead. AIDS continues to bring focus to the schisms and fractures in health and development.

Chapter 8
Funding the epidemic

The response to HIV and AIDS has to be funded, whether the emphasis is on prevention or treatment, or both. This disease is unique in part because of the complex financing. It also requires long-term commitment for those increasing numbers on relatively expensive lifesaving treatment. There are, of course, other diseases that require long-term care too such as diabetes and hypertension. The numbers requiring ART, their relative youth at initiation, and the cost of treatment, make AIDS different.

The history of funding

Initially AIDS was viewed primarily as a health concern for rich countries. Even after the acknowledgement that HIV was present in Africa and Asia, and that it spread through heterosexual transmission, the scale and potential impact was grossly underestimated. There was consequently little money allocated to the disease. In defence of early responses, it was neither clear where funds should be spent nor how much was needed. One of the early WHO interventions was to send out teams to countries to put in place standard short-term plans (STPs), which were, as the scale of the epidemic became apparent, replaced by medium-term plans (MTPs). These were limited, health-based, and relatively cheap.

The exceptions to this lack of funding were research and drug development costs incurred, mainly in the US, and to a lesser extent in France (Institute Pasteur in Paris) and in the UK (Wellcome Trust). In 1982, the US Congress allocated US$5 million to the Centers for Disease Control (CDC) for surveillance and another US$10 million to the National Institutes of Health (NIH) for research into the disease. In 1983, the first bill that sanctioned funding (US$12 million for the DHHS) specifically for AIDS research and treatment was passed. By 1985, US$70 million had been allocated for research, excluding resources mobilized in the private sector who, again, were primarily Western and American.

Why were money and people (especially scientists) allocated to this new problem so quickly in the West? The answer lies in the rapid mobilization of the gay community who set up AIDS-specific organizations even before the virus had been identified. In January 1982, the Gay Men's Health Crisis was established in New York City as a non-profit, volunteer-supported, and community-based AIDS service organization. When, in 1985, American actor Rock Hudson died of AIDS, he left US$250,000 to set up the American Foundation for AIDS Research (amfAR).

Lack of attention to the disease that was killing so many of their number, and slow progress in finding treatments, led the gay community to channel their anger and frustration in extraordinary and effective activism. ACT-UP, established in 1987, became an international advocacy group working for legislation, medical research, treatment, and policies to end AIDS.

The effectiveness of these articulate, organized activists, many from creative careers, in putting pressure on governments, scientists, and the pharmaceutical industry, cannot be overstated. The same level of political engagement around financial mobilization and drug prices was not seen in the resource-poor world, with the exception of the South African Treatment Action

Campaign (TAC) and in Brazil. The numerous grassroots and civil society organizations were more geared to providing support to patients, their families, and orphans.

In 1986, the US National Academy of Sciences issued a report critical of the government response, and called for a US$2 billion investment. In 1989, the Health Resources and Services Administration (HRSA) was granted US$20 million for HIV care and treatment through the Home-Based and Community-Based Care State Grant programme. In 1990, Congress enacted the Ryan White Comprehensive AIDS Resources Emergency (CARE) Act, providing US$220.5 million for HIV community-based care and treatment services in its first year alone. Ryan White was an Indiana teenager with haemophilia who acquired AIDS through contaminated blood products. Excluded from school, his plight became a focus for activism.

This pattern of expenditure on research, development, and support for those affected by AIDS was mirrored across the developed world, frequently with the impetus of activist engagement. It was not until the mid-1990s that the potential global impact of AIDS was acknowledged. Indeed there was active opposition to dealing with the disease. Epidemiologist Jonathan Mann founded the WHO's Global Programme for AIDS in 1986. By March 1990 he had resigned on principle to protest about the lack of UN response, in particular from the WHO Director-General Hiroshi Nakajima. That the WHO should be so short-sightedly unresponsive was unforgivable: tragically they were not alone in this failure.

In 1994, the UN finally acknowledged 'the magnitude and impact [of HIV/AIDS were] greatest in developing countries.' In 1996 UNAIDS was established under the leadership of Peter Piot in Geneva, with the mandate of coordinating the response of the UN agency co-sponsors and mobilizing the global response. Of especial significance for funding in the low- and middle-income countries were the January 2000 UN Security Council meeting, the MDGs, and the 2001 UNGASS Declaration.

Mobilizing international money

There was a time of plenty for the epidemic. The establishment of the Global Fund (GF) in 2002 began this trend, which is also shown in Figure 12. The first round of GF grants—worth US$378 million—were awarded to thirty-one countries in April 2002. The GF was established to respond to AIDS, TB, and malaria, and the distribution was 50 per cent for AIDS, 18 per cent for TB, and 32 per cent for malaria. This was maintained up to and during the 2014–16 allocation periods, and the split was reconfirmed at the GF board meeting in Geneva in November 2015.

GF funding was allocated to countries on the basis of detailed applications made in 'rounds', with deadlines for submissions. These were evaluated by independent panels. In 2014, the allocation method changed, and countries were given notional amounts they could apply for. There was some 'incentive' money for which countries could compete. The new funding model focused on countries with the highest burden and least ability to pay; offered predictable funding through the 'allocation amount'; actively supported applications to improve the success rates; and put in place a requirement for some level of domestic funding. The GF has mobilized large sums, but is a technical solution to a complex problem. The one area where success has been limited is in health systems strengthening.

The World Trade Organization's (WTO) Doha Declaration in November 2002, affirmed the rights of developing countries to buy or manufacture generic medications for public health crises, and AIDS was determined to be such a crisis. In the same year, the WHO issued its first guidelines for the use of ART in low-income settings.

12. Total resources for HIV/AIDS in low- and middle-income countries.

The subsequent agreement on Trade-Related Aspects of Intellectual Property Rights (TRIPS), provided an opportunity for poorer countries to expand access to low cost ART. This allowed production and importation of drugs in cheaper, generic forms. There is pressure on countries to limit use of TRIPS flexibility clauses, known as TRIPS-plus provisions, and adapt their laws to provide greater intellectual property protection and enforcement. This could cause prices to escalate.

The year 2002 also saw the establishment of the Clinton HIV/AIDS Initiative as part of the Clinton Foundation. This was a global organization committed to expanding access to care and treatment for HIV/AIDS, malaria, and TB, and for strengthening health systems. In 2010, the AIDS Initiative became a separate non-profit organization: the Clinton Health Access Initiative (CHAI).

The next major boost to funding was President Bush's creation of PEPFAR in 2003. This began as a US$15 billion, five-year plan to combat AIDS, primarily in countries with a high burden of infections. In March, the Bill and Melinda Gates Foundation (BMGF) awarded a US$60 million grant to the International Partnership for Microbicides to support research and development of microbicides to prevent transmission of HIV.

In 2006, UNITAID, a global health initiative, was established by Brazil, Chile, France, Norway, and the United Kingdom. It is hosted by the WHO in Geneva. Over twenty-five countries, and the BMGF, were UNITAID members by 2016. UNITAID looks for innovative interventions, as well as tackling inefficiencies in markets for medicines, diagnostics, and prevention for HIV and AIDS, malaria, and TB. Between 2007 and 2014, US$2.4 billion was raised of which 62 per cent came from a 'solidarity levy' on airline tickets (see the section on 'Domestic and innovative funding').

Global HIV and AIDS spending in the developing world and Eastern Europe increased from US$4.6 billion in 2003 to US$14.6 billion in 2008. At the end of that year, President Bush signed legislation reauthorizing PEPFAR for an additional five years for up to US$48 billion. The US contribution meant that, with the 2008 financial crash, AIDS funding flatlined rather than fell.

From 2008 onward, major shifts occurred in the global HIV and AIDS response. The financial crisis created uncertainty. The status of HIV and AIDS as a premier health threat was eroded. There was a shift from an emergency state to a normalization of the response, helped by the fact that, due to new drugs, HIV-infected people were living longer, more productive lives.

The United States accounts for the majority of bilateral and multilateral funding for global HIV and AIDS responses (64.5 per cent from the United States, followed by 12.9 per cent from the UK, 3.7 per cent from France, 3.2 per cent from Germany, and 2.5 per cent from the Netherlands). Since 2006, these countries have accounted for roughly 80 per cent of all HIV funding from donor governments. Bilateral funding provided over 70 per cent of HIV funding from donors in 2014.

In 2014, 27 per cent of international HIV assistance was provided through multilateral organizations such as the Global Fund, UNITAID, and other United Nations agencies. Six donor governments provided the majority of their HIV funding through the Global Fund (Canada, the European Commission, France, Germany, Italy, and Japan). Private philanthropies provided US$592 million for global HIV and AIDS programmes in 2013. The Bill and Melinda Gates Foundation is the leading philanthropic funder of international HIV efforts. To date, the foundation has provided more than US$2.5 billion towards tackling the global HIV epidemic and has given an additional US$1.4 billion to the Global Fund.

Taking stock

At the end of 2015, total investments in the AIDS response in low- and middle-income countries totalled US$21.7 billion. This almost met the investment target set in the 2011 Declaration: mobilizing between US$22 billion and US$24 billion by 2015. It is quite remarkable so much money was raised from such a variety of sources.

The financial mobilization has not been unproblematic. AIDS was, correctly, treated as an exceptional global challenge. Its champions in the early years were articulate and outraged. The argument that this exceptional disease needed an exceptional response was accepted in the West. The result was that funding came from international sources. In some countries, over 95 per cent of funding was external. According to a 2015 *Lancet* article, in Tanzania in 2011 only 1.2 per cent of the AIDS spending came from government, external expenditure on AIDS was US$432 million with government spending just US$8 million. In Zambia two years later in 2013, only 10.6 per cent came from government.

The international contribution led to a lack of local ownership and a dependency mind-set. A review of twelve PEPFAR countries by Results for Development noted: 'deeply ingrained perceptions by finance and other senior government officials that donors will take care of the AIDS programme', as indeed donors have done over the past decade. This gave rise to low domestic allocations, little local involvement, and an abnegation of responsibility in some countries. Donor-determined strategies and priorities might not reflect local needs or conditions. A prime example was the abstinence 'earmark' by the US government, where a proportion of US money had to be spent on promoting abstinence.

Since international funding went to marginal groups like IDUs in Russia, MSMs in a number of African countries, and support services for sex workers in many locations, governments ignored these populations, allowing donors to take care of their needs. Doubtless support went to key populations who otherwise would have been neglected, but the question is: where does government responsibility begin and end?

The influx of money led to vertical programmes or 'stovepipes'. The funding was for specific diseases as opposed to the broader health system. The advantage of this for the donors was twofold: firstly, the money was easier to track; secondly, the results were more easily attributed to their interventions. Unfortunately, it was not always what the recipient countries needed or would have prioritized and led to waste and duplication.

In 2016 health funding in most low- and middle-income countries was through government budgets fed from general tax revenues. HIV and AIDS have been the exception. The global trend is towards universal health care (UHC) in various forms. This is more appropriate for mainstreaming and normalizing AIDS. UHC would be expected to include ART and possibly prevention activities. In Thailand in 2006, the ART programme was transferred to the UHC scheme which covered 98 per cent of its population.

Looking forward

AIDS resource needs are projected to increase at least until 2020. A 2015 modelling study by Atun and others suggests that, in sub-Saharan Africa, the total resources required for HIV prevention and treatment from 2015 to 2050 range from US$110 billion to US$293 billion, depending on treatment and prevention scenarios. For example, in order to maintain current coverage levels for treatment and prevention, with eligibility for treatment initiation at CD4 count of $< 500/mm^3$, the total cost to 2050 is US$110 billion. If treatment is extended to all HIV+ individuals and prevention scaled up, the total cost to 2050 would be around US$293 billion.

The UNAIDS 'Fast-Track Approach' argues scaling the response up by 2020 would prevent infections, save lives, and ultimately require less money. The view from Geneva is that the world has limited time to make these investments. They estimated current investments were close to US$22 billion in 2015. Another US$8 to US$12 billion would allow the fast-track goals to be met. Their strategy will require US$31 billion in 2020. The argument that frontloading would work is undoubtedly sensible, especially for successful prevention. The unspoken assumption is that the interventions will work as well as projected.

Some innovative thinking came from the RUSH Foundation's RethinkHIV consortium of researchers who looked at evidence related to the costs, benefits, effects, fiscal implications, and developmental impacts of HIV interventions in sub-Saharan Africa. The title of the 2015 roundtable event in Boston, 'From a Death Sentence to a Debt Sentence: Meeting the Challenge of Long-term Liabilities of HIV Funding', succinctly encapsulates the essential issue. Providing ART is an irreversible commitment across the lifetime of the person living with HIV. Almost all of the costs lie in the future: putting someone on treatment incurs a liability similar to a debt. These debts are not currently 'on the books' and remain unacknowledged by governments and donors. 'There is a disturbing disconnect between short-term funding cycles and long-term financial liabilities, as well as accountability for these between donors and affected governments.'

The global economic downturn and a climate of austerity mean Development Assistance for Health (DAH) has plateaued and is unlikely to increase in the near future. Traditional donor countries face their own challenges. There is concern over the ever-present threat of new diseases (or the re-emergence of old diseases—e.g. Ebola in 2014). The reality is that global development assistance will remain static, since any new money will go to environmental issues, which are now at the top of the global agenda. While health exponents advocate for increased assistance, it won't materialize from traditional sources unless convincing new arguments are found.

Domestic and innovative funding

While the total global spending on HIV and AIDS grew significantly, the share of external funding declined from 60 per cent in 2008 to 43 per cent in 2014. The GF and PEPFAR are looking to see increased local ownership—in the case of PEPFAR they plan to transition out of countries. Some countries have made significant progress; South Africa has the largest resource need for HIV and AIDS and contributes approximately 82 per cent from the domestic budget.

Between 2009 and 2014, eighty-four out of 121 low- and middle-income countries increased domestic AIDS spending. Of these countries, forty-six reported an increase of more than 50 per cent, including thirty-five countries that increased in domestic spending by more than 100 per cent. High increases in the percentage may be the result of low initial levels. If a country allocated US$100 to HIV/AIDS in 2009 but US$200 by 2014, that would be a 100 per cent increase. Indeed in sub-Saharan Africa, the Democratic Republic of the Congo, Gambia, Liberia, and Zimbabwe, reported more than 100 per cent increases between 2009 and 2014, off very low bases.

Economic growth and new revenue sources will increase the fiscal space for health spending. As countries progress and incomes grow, HIV will be concentrated in middle-income countries, which will receive less donor support and may face higher prices.

The question is what to do in poor countries with a low GDP per capita and high HIV prevalence. Malawi, Mozambique, Uganda, Zimbabwe, Lesotho, and Zambia all have prevalence over 10 per cent and per capita GDPs of less than US$3,000. Malawi is the worst case: the GDP per capita is US$255 and the government health expenditure per capita is only US$26. Clearly the AIDS programmes will remain dependent on donor input for the foreseeable future.

Innovative funding may generate potential new finance. From 2002 to 2012, more than US$6 billion was raised internationally by innovative financing instruments. For example, Ghana's National Health Insurance Levy added 2.5 per cent to VAT. The revenue generated by this tax was used to fund approximately 70 per cent of the National Health Insurance Scheme, a fund designed to reduce financial barriers to health care. In Thailand, a consumption tax on alcohol and tobacco earmarked 2 per cent of the revenue generated to go to the Thai Health Promotion Foundation. Almost US$60 million has been generated and spent on health promotion. Zimbabwe's National AIDS Trust was set up in 1999 to fund the National AIDS Council (NAC) and reduce its reliance on external funding. This 3 per cent levy generated US$2.6 billion between 2000, when it began operating, and 2006, and in 2011, US$26 million was collected.

Kenya established a High Level Steering Committee for Sustainable HIV Financing which pools additional public and private resources. They have allocated between 0.5 and 1 per cent of government revenues to a Trust Fund which will also be financed by other sources (such as an airline levy). It has been estimated this will fill 70 per cent of the HIV funding gap between 2010 and 2020, and 159 per cent between 2020 and 2030.

A number of earmarked special taxes have been used and others are being considered. These include financial and currency transactions, which are levies placed on specific monetary transactions. There is currently no example of these taxes being used for health services. Versions of employment levies based on Zimbabwe's levy are being considered in other settings but there is no evidence yet of them being implemented. Air ticket taxes have raised money for UNITAID. Nine countries have since implemented these: Cameroon, Chile, Congo, France, Madagascar,

Mali, Mauritius, Niger, and the Republic of Korea. The ticket levy is described on the UNITAID web site as: 'A painless addition to the cost of a ticket, the levy is a leading example of globalisation working for the poor.'

Mobile phone levies are reported from Rwanda and Uganda: a consumption tax. Earmarked taxes on alcohol and tobacco (sin taxes), have a great deal of potential in mobilizing and sustaining resources to health and changing behaviours. The question is whether HIV, and even health, is the priority of the ministry of finance once the money is collected.

Other funding sources suggested include concessionary loans for HIV and AIDS programmes; debt conversion (known also 'debt2health'); AIDS lotteries; utilizing dormant funds (e.g. property which is unclaimed); social impact bonds; social development bonds; diaspora bonds; a micro-levy on extractive industries; sovereign bonds securitized against future revenue streams; and special fundraising such as the existing GF Product Red, a brand where partner companies such as Nike, Apple Inc., Coca-Cola Company, and Starbucks brand a product with the Product Red logo and 50 per cent of the profit generated is donated to the GF.

Innovative funding is notoriously unreliable. Schemes may not work, be as lucrative as expected, or be allocated to intended targets. Innovative financing mechanisms are not the 'magic bullet' that will end development's funding woes. Most are still in their infancy, and success has not yet been seen. There is concern that innovative financing mechanisms may be used to justify replacing (or decreasing) DAH and domestic budgetary commitments.

Efficiency savings in health systems could theoretically create substantial fiscal space, achieving higher HIV treatment and prevention coverage without requiring budgetary increases. The

International Monetary Fund (IMF) estimates that as much as 50 per cent of health expenditures in low- and middle-income countries may be wasted or inefficiently used. Better health care system design and financing may improve the efficiency of global resource use. In South Africa in 2010, bound by the terms of its existing tender for ARTs, the government only bought one-third of its products at internationally competitive prices. Over the following two years there was a 53 per cent reduction in the cost of ART drugs, with savings of US$640 million.

Security is crucial

In AIDS we can plot the trajectory of epidemic. This includes the demographic and social impact, the epidemiology, and resource requirements needed to control, maintain, and ultimately end this disease. What is required is an upfront commitment led by governments where the epidemic is an issue. Funding from international organizations and NGOs will be useful in subsidizing the costs of the HIV/AIDS response, but they are finite resources shared by many needy countries and other causes.

A report funded by USAID on financing ART in low- and middle-income countries articulated the issue. The ability of a country to finance HIV and AIDS depends on the wealth of the country and the distribution of the wealth; the cost of the ART programme; and the willingness of the country (government, private sector, and people) to allocate funds to ART. As the authors noted the wealth of a country is hard to affect, but economies are growing. The distribution of wealth can be influenced but is a general political decision. The cost of an ART programme depends on prioritization, cost-effectiveness, and efficiency. The crucial question is the degree to which a country will allocate resources. However, if people are put on ART, then this is a long-term commitment that requires timely and predictable funding flows.

Chapter 9
Big issues and major challenges

If a third edition of this Very Short Introduction to HIV and AIDS were produced in 2022, it would be a different book to this one. By then, unless something dramatic happens (e.g. an unforeseen mutation of the virus into a more virulent variety), the epidemic will be under control across the world. The number of new infections will continue to fall; there will be virtually no vertical transmission from mothers to infants; and for those who have the misfortune to be infected, treatment will be monthly pills or implants, increasingly effective and simple, with fewer side effects.

The prevention armamentarium will include microbicides accepted and used by women, medical male circumcision will be widespread, and it is to be hoped that neonatal circumcision will be routine. It is unlikely there will be a vaccine or cure, but both will be closer.

AIDS will not end in 2030 as UNAIDS has hoped. There will still be some new infections. If, as expected, we are successful at putting people on treatment, there will be significant numbers living with HIV and taking the drugs. These will be people who have been infected from the turn of the millennium on, although many of them will, of course, be ageing. Indeed AIDS and the elderly may become an important topic for research.

A next edition of the VSI would be a history that looks at the rise and fall of AIDS as a public health catastrophe. It would ask questions about why the epidemic took hold, what drove the responses, and why it proved so hard to eliminate from the world. It would trace the rise of UNAIDS and the GF. It would look at how their missions changed and how they adapted (or possibly closed). However, there are still a number of big issues and these are addressed later in this chapter.

Location and population

The full name of the UNAIDS World AIDS Day report in 2015 was: 'On the Fast-Track to End AIDS by 2030: Focus on Location and Populations'. It was significant for two major reasons. Firstly, it called for the end of AIDS by 2030, in line with the SDGs, and acknowledged that for this to happen, major investments and initiatives are required over the next five years. In their terminology the response must be frontloaded! The Kenyan case, where there are 1.4 million people living with HIV, is the example used to illustrate this. Business as usual, with a US$1 billion investment over thirty years, will prevent 1.1 million new infections; frontloading will mean 22 per cent more infections will be averted, and consequently less health care and treatment will be required in the years ahead. Secondly, the report recognized the need to focus on specific areas and populations. Again Kenya provides an example: 65 per cent of new infections took place in just nine of the forty-seven administrative counties. Prevalence was highest among sex workers at 29 per cent; MSM and IDU prevalence were both 18 per cent. It makes sense for the resources and efforts to be focused on these counties and people.

Unusually for a UN-produced document, the report talked about what was not working in the response. This included: providing wrong services defined as misusing resources and not to scaling up the most cost-effective interventions in local contexts; working in the wrong places (in locations where there is not an epidemic);

reaching the wrong people (those who are not at risk and ignoring those with the greatest need); and doing things in the wrong way (not procuring ART in a cost-effective manner).

A major stumbling block they identify is resistance to change from leaders—even when the information is available. The report notes: 'Moving forward, national and local leaders must make tough decisions about reallocating resources according to the results of these efficiency analyses'. These analyses have and are being conducted with UNAIDS's support. Practically, this means taking resources away from low-burden districts or regions, and reallocating them to areas of high burden. It will mean paying especial attention to stigmatized populations, those who politicians most times would rather ignore.

The 'business as usual' approach to AIDS programmes will not, UNAIDS warned, be enough to even maintain existing gains. In Zimbabwe, the investment scenarios showed that annual new infections would double between 2015 and 2025, and that AIDS deaths would increase by a third if the programmes simply continue as before. If on the other hand there was better focus, then gains could be made. In Zimbabwe, between October 2013 and September 2014, 80 per cent of new HIV diagnoses were identified at 30 per cent of the 1,724 PEPFAR-supported sites. Forty-nine sites did not identify any cases and there were fewer than four at 123 sites. Clearly there is a need to provide education and prevention activities across the country. There must be surveillance and monitoring in order to ensure there is not an outbreak in any location, but interventions should be fit for purpose.

The issues of stigma and discrimination need to be addressed. Even in high-prevalence Swaziland, where AIDS is a part of life, 37.4 per cent per cent of women and 36.2 per cent of men aged 15 to 49 expressed discriminatory attitudes towards people living with HIV. Across the world, same-sex acts are illegal in seventy-eight countries, with the possibility of the death penalty being imposed in five. Reaching MSMs in these contexts becomes very difficult. Drug use is generally criminalized (use may be allowed in some countries, but trafficking is a criminal offence everywhere). In Indonesia, where 56.4 per cent of IDUs in Jakarta are HIV+, many drug-related offences carry the death penalty. At the most basic level, stigma may discourage people from obtaining, carrying, or using condoms. At its most extreme stigma has been recorded to be so damaging as to compromise ART adherence: people don't want to be seen taking tablets.

In the developed world, an innovation in AIDS prevention is PrEP. The problem is this might encourage people to engage in unsafe sex and, while they are protected against HIV transmission, other sexually transmitted infections will continue to be a risk. It may be that this intervention can and should be targeted to particular high-risk pools of people such as sex workers in impoverished countries. Alternatively PrEP might be something that can be socially marketed.

Technology

The rise of new technologies is both a blessing and a curse for the AIDS epidemic. The ability to link over the Internet or smart phones to arrange casual sexual encounters has been a major new development. The use of these apps is not confined to Western countries. They can be accessed where people have smart phones. The prevention responses lag behind these innovations. There needs to be some serious consideration about changing patterns of sexuality. Phones can be used to send messages, ranging from ones concerning safety in clubs to reminders to take drugs. There are a range of companies and entrepreneurs engaged in eHealth, an area of innovation to track as it is one of the waves of the future.

The proliferation of GPS allows the epidemic to be mapped; handheld computers enable data to be collected; and new techniques allow ever more granular analysis. The importance of data is recognized by all the donors and increasingly by governments. It can be particularly helpful with supply chain management. Early warning systems can be set up to ensure ART supplies are available and warn when they are running low.

Technology has an important role to play in the development of new and better drugs, and in increasing the availability of and speed of testing. In the United States testing in community pharmacies has been piloted. In Malawi a feasibility study showed self-testing, where a person can use a rapid diagnostic kit and get the result in private, was successful. Three-quarters of people who were given a kit used it, and 76 per cent of these then accessed a counsellor to talk about the results. This enabled those who were infected to be put on care while it provided an incentive to those who were not infected to stay that way. The fifth wave of public health, the culture for health, is emerging and is driven by personal technologies.

Reaching adolescent girls and young women

In Africa the majority of infections are among this group. The challenges are many: patriarchal, exploitative, and disrespectful attitudes towards young women and girls are a major issue. Intimate partner violence and lack of access to opportunities help drive the epidemic. Poverty and food insecurity may lead to higher levels of transactional sex. It is not enough to provide prevention technology such as condoms or microbicides; these women need to be empowered to make decisions about their own health.

The structural barriers have to be addressed. There have been, and continue to be, pilot projects examining conditional cash transfers which might, among other things, keep girls in school. This is known to be protective against HIV transmission. In Botswana the length of schooling was increased by one year in 1996 which was found to increase the likelihood of young women remaining HIV–. The challenge is to move from pilot projects to national ones. The role of social security is something that needs further analysis.

A major new initiative in ten countries in Eastern and Southern Africa known as: 'DREAMS: Determined, Resilient, Empowered, AIDS-Free, Mentored and Safe Women', is being supported by PEPFAR, the BMGF, and an NGO called Girl Effect. This not only provides HIV services, but is designed to address the structural drivers that increase HIV risk. DREAMS is being integrated into local systems and targeted so as to not duplicate existing programmes. If this project works, then the potential for it to be expanded is considerable.

Women and men have to be discouraged from transactional and intergenerational sex, and that means women need resources, and men need to show respect and care. One effective advertisement was a billboard near the University Campus in Swaziland. It showed an older man in a smart new car talking to (chatting up, by implication and body language) a young woman who was leaning into the window. 'How would you feel if this was your daughter?' asked the caption.

Finance

The reality is that AIDS is expensive. One of the encouraging steps taken in the past decade is to recognize that putting people on treatment will help prevent the transmission of the virus. This has led to a global policy seeking to treat all newly identified HIV cases immediately. The treatment cascades show us that the challenge is to identify HIV+ people, link them to care, have them initiate treatment, and be adherent. Only once all these criteria are met will they become and remain virally suppressed. It is unfortunately not simple.

In many poorer nations, choices have to be made about where to spend government budgets. AIDS is just one of a number of health challenges faced by citizens and ministries of health. What is different though is that prevention ensures that future treatment costs will not have to be met.

The question of who bears the burden of the epidemic needs more thought and attention. The activist community was articulate and Western. They called for action in their own countries and then looked globally. AIDS was a solidarity movement.

The world has changed and AIDS is no longer prioritized as it once was. There is no doubt that in the early years there was good reason to be extremely concerned. The success of many interventions changed the threat level, and while efforts need to be constantly evaluated and updated regionally and globally, it is time to reassess the epidemic and how we respond to it. HIV has not gone away, but rather it has found a home primarily among the poor and the marginalized. The question at each level, national and international, is how much do we value the lives of these people? The problem is the long-term liability may be too great for a number of countries.

Tipping points

Even ten years ago it was hard to predict the tipping points in the AIDS epidemic. In hindsight, they were the discovery of treatment and the establishment of UNAIDS in 1996; the Durban AIDS Conference in 2000; the setting up of the GF in 2002 and PEPFAR in 2003; and the TRIPS agreement in 2002. Most recently the new SDGs could be seen as a negative tipping point since the disease no longer features prominently as it did in the MDGs.

Today there is ample reason to be optimistic. The success in prevention, the amazing advances in treatment, and continued scientific research are all encouraging. Unfortunately there needs to be continued vigilance. The scientists working on treatments have, on a number of occasions, believed they cured patients, only to find the virus had become dormant, remaining in locations in the body that drugs could not reach. The same is true on a global scale. The AIDS movement transformed the health care system with increasing emphasis on community services and task shifting. It also led to empowerment of individuals with HIV who took control of their health and played a role in managing it, a new kind of 'patient', but this has been more a Western phenomenon than a worldwide one.

In order to find and eliminate HIV conclusively, we need to address the poor and marginal groups, and that means understanding the determinants of health. AIDS was the disease of the last two decades of the 20th century. Getting to grips with it will be the story of the first two decades of the 21st century.

References and further reading

AIDS is the most studied disease in human history. The literature is huge, ranging from dense scientific writing to popular texts. In addition there are theses, press clippings, and the Internet. Over the past thirty years I have read widely on the subject, reflecting on the rich diversity of information and ideas I have accessed. The bibliography represents a small part of what is available.

General literature and data

The World Wide Web provides the best source of up-to-date information. The prime websites are: UNAIDS <www.unaids.org> (where the Global AIDS Epidemic reports are accessible); the World Health Organisation <www.who.org>; UNDP <www.undp.org>; UNICEF <www.unicef.org>; the Global Fund for AIDS, TB and Malaria <www.theglobalfund.org>; the US Centres for Disease Control <www.cdc.gov>; and the World Bank <www.worldbank.org>. A good history is found on <www.avert.org>—an AIDS charity.

My work at HEARD from 1997 to 2013 can be accessed on <www.heard.org.za> and more recent publications either on <www.balsilliesschool.ca> or my own website <www.alan-whiteside.com>.

My co-authored book, Tony Barnett and Alan Whiteside, *AIDS in the Twenty-First Century: Disease and Globalisation* (2nd edn) (Palgrave, 2006) provided the early thinking. Recent general texts I would recommend are C. Timberg and D. Halperin, *Tinderbox: How the West Sparked the AIDS Epidemic and How the World Can Finally Overcome*

It (Penguin Books, 2013); Norman Fowler, *AIDS: Don't Die of Prejudice* (Backbite Publishing, 2014); and Peter Piot's biography, *No Time to Lose: A Life in Pursuit of Deadly Viruses* (WW Norton and company, 2012). Slightly old but still useful is Salim Karim and Quarraisha Karim (eds), *HIV/AIDS in South Africa* (Cambridge University Press, 2010). Janet Seeley's *HIV and East Africa: Thirty Years in the Shadow of an Epidemic* (Routledge, 2014) is outstanding.

Without a doubt the most sobering reflection on what pandemic disease can do to a society is Charles C. Mann, *Ancient Americans: Rewriting the History of the New World* (Granta Books, 2005).

Thought-provoking books are Alex de Waal, *AIDS and Power: Why There Is No Political Crisis—Yet* (Zed Books, 2006); and Stephen Lewis, *Race Against Time* (House of Anansi Press, 2005).

Chapter 1: The emergence and state of the HIV and AIDS epidemic

Excellent historical accounts of the disease include Randy Shilts, *And the Band Played On: Politics, People and the AIDS Epidemic* (St Martin's Press, 1987). Also of value is John Iliffe, *The African AIDS Epidemic: A History* (James Currey, 2006).

The original reports of the epidemic came from the 'United States Centers for Disease Control Morbidity and Mortality Weekly Report' (5 June 1981).

The data on the global epidemic is derived from the UNAIDS website, <www.unaids.org>.

The South African data and Figure 3 come from O. Shisana, T. Rehle, L. Simbayi, et al., 'South African National HIV Prevalence, Incidence and Behaviour Survey 2012' (Cape Town) and their earlier reports. The data on Europe comes from <https://www.gov.uk/government/organisations/public-health-england> and from the United States website <http://www.usphs.gov/>. Swaziland data are from G. Bicego et al., 'Recent Patterns in Population-Based HIV Prevalence in Swaziland', *PLoS ONE* (October 2013), DOI: 10.1371/journal.pone.0077101.

The Global Burden of Disease data is sourced from the IHME at <http://www.healthdata.org/gbd>.

The most useful work on zoonotic disease was D. Quammen, *Spillover: Animal Infections and the Next Human Pandemic* (WW Norton, 2013).

Chapter 2: How HIV and AIDS work and scientific responses

Trying to understanding the virus is not undertaken lightly. Useful books are Barry D. Schoub, *AIDS and HIV in Perspective: A Guide to Understanding the Virus and its Consequences* (2nd edn) (Cambridge University Press, 1999); Michael B.A. Oldstone, *Viruses, Plagues and History* (Oxford University Press, 2000); and Jaap Goudsmit, *Viral Sex* (Oxford University Press, 1998).

The issue of HIV and TB is important, and helpful articles were by Yan Wang, Charles Collins, Mercy Vergis, Nancy Gerein, and Jean Macq, 'HIV/AIDS and TB: Contextual Issues and Policy Choice in Programme Relations', *Tropical Medicine and International Health* 12(2) (February 2007); and N.R. Gandhi et al., 'Extensively Drug-Resistant Tuberculosis as a Cause of Death in Patients Co-Infected with Tuberculosis and HIV in a Rural Area of South Africa', *Lancet*, 368(9547) (November 2006). In addition updates came from the websites.

The early work on circumcision was from John C. Caldwell et al. (eds), 'Resistances to Behavioural Change to Reduce HIV/AIDS Infection', Health Transition Centre, Australian National University (1989). Also valuable was J.C. Caldwell, 'Lack of Male Circumcision and AIDS in Sub-Saharan Africa: Resolving the Conflict', National Center for Epidemiology and Population Health, The Australian National University (April 1995): 113–17.

The figures are adapted from R.A. Royce, A. Seña, W. Cates, and M.S.N. Cohen, 'Current Concepts: Sexual Transmission of HIV', *New England Journal of Medicine* 336 (10 April 1997): 1072–8.

Most of the data on Table 3 come from <http://www.cdc.gov/hiv/policies/law/risk.html>.

For information on vaccines, see <www.iavi.org>; for microbicides, see <www.ipm-microbicides.org>. The discussion on the treatment as prevention has generated numerous article but a good starting point is <http://www.aidsmap.com/The-HPTN-052-study/page/1847774/>.

Chapter 3: What shapes epidemics?

The discussion of AIDS nutrition and poverty is captured by Eileen Stillwaggon, *AIDS and the Ecology of Poverty* (Oxford University Press, 2006). The role of malaria was assessed by Laith J. Abu-Raddad, Padmaja Patnaik, and James G. Kublin, 'Dual Infection with HIV and Malaria Fuels the Spread of Both Diseases in Sub-Saharan Africa', *Science* (8 December 2006). The information on Ebola came from websites and news reports, the best being the WHO which also provided regular updates.

Interesting writing on sexual behaviours is taken from Soori Nnko, J. Ties Boerma, Mark Urassa, Gabriel Mwaluko, and Basia Zaba, 'Secretive Females or Swaggering Males? An Assessment of the Quality of Sexual Partnership Reporting in Rural Tanzania', Population Center, University of North Carolina at Chapel Hill (2002), retrieved from: <http://www.cpc.unc.edu/measure/resources/publications/wp-02-57?searchterm=swagger>.

The only meta-analysis of sexual behaviour data comes from Kaye Wellings, Martine Collumbien, Emma Slaymaker, Susheela Singh, Zoé Hodges, Dhaval Patel, and Nathalie Bajos, 'Sexual Behaviour in Context: A Global Perspective', *Lancet* (11 November 2006). Data are also drawn from the Durex Global Sex Survey, <www.durex.com>; and the Demographic and Health Surveys, <http://www.measuredhs.com/>.

The data on respondents in Nairobi comes from C. Timberg and D. Halperin, *Tinderbox: How the West Sparked the AIDS Epidemic and How the World Can Finally Overcome It* (Penguin Books, 2013).

The seminal article on concurrency of partnering is Daniel T. Halperin and Helen Epstein, 'Concurrent Sexual Partnerships Help to Explain Africa's High HIV Prevalence: Implications for Prevention', *Lancet* 364(9428) (3–9 July 2004): 4–6.

The model showing impact of focused intervention in Kenya is from the World Bank, 'Confronting AIDS: Public Priorities in a Global Epidemic', A World Bank Policy Research Report, Oxford University Press for the World Bank, European Commission and UNAIDS, (1997).

An attempt to identify the drivers of the epidemic in Swaziland is Alan Whiteside, Catarina Andrade, Lisa Arrehag, Solomon Dlamini, Themba Ginindza, and Anokhi Parikh, 'The Socio-Economic Impact of HIV/AIDS in Swaziland', HIV AIDS Economic Research Division and NERCHA (2006), <www.heard.org.za>.

The data on sexual violence are from the WHO, 'Violence against Women: Intimate Partner and Sexual Violence against Women,' retrieved from <http://www.who.int/mediacentre/factsheets/fs239/en/>.

Chapter 4: Illness, death, and the demographic impact

The information on vital registration is from World Bank Group, 'Global Civil Registration and Vital Statistics: Scaling up Investment Plan 2015–2024', World Bank & WHO, retrieved from <http://www-wds.worldbank.org/external/default/WDSContentServer/WDSP/IB/2014/05/28/000456286_20140528170841/Rendered/PDF/883510WP0CRVS000Box385194B00PUBLIC0.pdf> (May 2014).

The United States mortality data are from CDC, 'HIV in the United States: At a Glance', retrieved from <http://www.cdc.gov/hiv/statistics/basics/ataglance.html>.

The best writing on the Mbeki era comes from Nicoli Nattrass's two books: *Mortal Combat: AIDS Denialism and the Struggle for Antiretrovirals in South Africa* (University of KwaZulu-Natal Press, 2007); and *The AIDS Conspiracy: Science Fights Back* (Columbia University Press, 2012).

All the South African data come from Statistics South Africa, 'Mortality and Causes of Death in South Africa, 2013: Findings from Death Notification', retrieved from <http://www.statssa.gov.za/publications/P03093/P030932013.pdf>.

Demographic data are drawn from the websites of U.S. Census Bureau, 'The AIDS Pandemic in the 21st Century' (U.S. Government Printing Office, 2004); 'International Population Reports' <http://www.unfpa.org/swop>; the United Nations Population Division, Department of Economic and Social Affairs <http://www.un.org/en/development/desa/population/>; and the WHO Global Health Observatory <http://www.who.int/gho/en/>.

The South African data are from Statistics South Africa, 'Mortality and Causes of Death 2013', *Statistics SA* (February 2013).

The 2014 Swaziland Multiple Indicator Cluster Survey key findings came from <https://mics-surveys-prod.s3.amazonaws.com/MICS5/Eastern%20and%20Southern%20Africa/Swaziland/2014/Key%20findings/Swaziland%202014%20MICS%20KFR_English.pdf>.

The article on the effect of a mother's death was by Marie-Louse Newell, Heena Brahmbatt, and Peter H. Ghys 'Child Mortality and HIV Infection in Africa', *AIDS* 18(2) (June 2004).

Data on life expectancy, IMR, and CMR are drawn from the World Bank's interactive data set: <http://data.worldbank.org/>.

Other data come from UNAIDS, 'How AIDS Changed Everything. MDG 6: 15 Years, 15 Lessons of Hope from the AIDS Response', *UNAIDS*, p. 113, retrieved from <http://www.unaids.org/sites/default/files/media_asset/MDG6Report_en.pdf>; and the United Nations Population Division, 'Population and HIV/AIDS 2010', retrieved from <http://www.un.org/en/development/desa/population/publications/pdf/hiv/populationAndHIVAIDS2010.pdf>.

The first of the Botswana population pyramids is from the US Bureau of the Census, the second from: <http://www.indexmundi.com/botswana/age_structure.html>.

The two recent books that touch on orphaning are J. Seeley, *HIV and East Africa: Thirty Years in the Shadow of the Epidemic* (Routledge, 2013); and M. Chazan, *The Grandmother's Movement: Solidarity and Survival in the Time of AIDS* (McGill-Queens University Press, 2015).

The Actuarial Society of South Africa has data and models at <www.actuarialsociety.org.za>.

Chapter 5: Production and people

The GDP data come from the World Bank retrieved from: <http://data.worldbank.org/indicator/NY.GDP.PCAP.CD>.

The new book is M. Haacker, *The Economics of the Global Response to HIV/AIDS* (Oxford University Press, 2016).

The concept of moral duty is from P. Collier, O. Sterck, and R. Manning, 'The Moral and Fiscal Implications of Anti-Retroviral Therapies for HIV in Africa', CSAE Working Paper (February 2015).

The best empirical work on HIV and AIDS and production comes from the Center for International Health and Development at Boston University, four papers need specific reference. They are: Sydney Rosen, Rich Feeley, Patrick Connelly, and Jonathon Simon, 'The Private Sector and HIV/AIDS in Africa: Taking Stock of Six Years of Applied Research', Health and Development Discussion Paper No. 7 (June 2006); M. Fox, S. Rosen, W. MacLeod, M. Wasunna, M. Bii, G. Foglia, and J. Simon, 'The Impact of HIV/AIDS on Labour Productivity in Kenya', *Tropical Medicine and International Health* 9 (2004): 318–24; Bruce Larson, Petan Hamazakaza, Crispin Kapunda, Coillard Hamusimbi, and Sydney Rosen, *Morbidity, Mortality, and Crop Production: An Empirical Study of Smallholder Cotton Growing Households in the Central Province of Zambia* (Center for International Health and Development, 2004); and Frank Feeley, Maggie Banda, Sydney Rosen, and Matthew Fox, *The Impact of HIV/AIDS on the Judicial System in the Republic of Zambia* (Center for Global Health & Development, 2006). Their most recent relevant work is B.A. Larson et al. 'Antiretroviral Therapy, Labor Productivity, and Sex: A Longitudinal Cohort Study of Tea Pluckers in Kenya', *AIDS* 27(1) (January 2013): 115–23. All available from the CIHD website <http://sph.bu.edu/index.php?option=com_content&task=view&id=427&Itemid=526>.

The business and AIDS websites are Global Business Coalition on HIV/AIDS, Tuberculosis and Malaria retrieved from <http://www.gbchealth.org/>.

South African Business Coalition on Health and Aids retrieved from <http://www.sabcoha.org>.

The information on fish production in Lake Malawi comes from a news report by R. Mweninguwe, 'Hot Business in Need of Water', *Development and Cooperation* (January 2013) retrieved from <http://www.dandc.eu/en/article/fish-farming-has-become-indispensible-malawi-industry-affected-climate-change-induced-water>.

In the discussion on AIDS and agriculture the 'new variant famine' ideas were published in Alex De Waal and Alan Whiteside, 'New Variant Famine: AIDS and Food Crisis in Southern Africa', *Lancet* 362(9391) (11 October 2003): 1234–7. The Malawi data comes from Anne C. Conroy, Malcolm J. Blackie, Alan Whiteside, Justin C. Malewezi, and Jeffrey D. Sachs, *Poverty, AIDS and Hunger: Breaking the Poverty Trap in Malawi* (Palgrave, 2006), while that for Zimbabwe is from P. Kwaramba, 'The Socio-economic Impact of HIV/AIDS on Communal Agricultural Production Systems in Zimbabwe', Economic Advisory Project, Friedrich Ebert Stiftung, Harare (1998), Working Paper 19; and The Famine Early Warning Network, <www.fews.net>. The follow-up paper is by Michael Loevinsohn, 'The 2001–03 Famine and the Dynamics of HIV in Malawi: A Natural Experiment', *PLoS ONE* (September 2015) DOI: 10.1371/journal.pone.0135108.

The work on grandmothers and Warwick Junction is drawn from May Chazan's ethnographic research presented at the International AIDS Conference in Toronto (2006), 'What Will Happen When Grandmothers Die? Unpacking the Gender and Generational Implications of Aids and Household Changes among Street Traders in Durban', South Africa (Abstract WEAD0101).

Chapter 6: Development, numbers, and politics

The initial thinking on the Human Development Index comes from the UNDP, 'Human Development Report 1990' (Oxford University Press, 1990), p. 40, retrieved from <http://hdr.undp.org/sites/default/files/reports/219/hdr_1990_en_complete_nostats.pdf>.

Subsequent data are drawn from the UNDP website, <www.undp.org>.

The information on the United Nations, 'Sustainable Development Goals' was retrieved from <https://sustainabledevelopment.un.org/?menu=1300>.

The explanation for PEPFAR comes from G.W. Bush, 'Better Health Care in Africa Must Go Beyond HIV', *TIME* (October 2015) retrieved from <http://time.com/4065971/george-w-bush-health-care-africa/>.

The data on PEPFAR especially the funding and results come from their website at: <http://www.pepfar.gov/funding/index.htm>.

The links between AIDS and conflict were postulated by among others Martin Schönteich, 'Age and AIDS: South Africa's Crime Time Bomb', *AIDS Analysis Africa* 10(2) (August/September 1999); and countered by Laurie Garrett, 'HIV and National Security: Where are the Links? A Council on Foreign Relations Report' (2005); Alan Whiteside, Alex de Waal, and Tsadkan Gebre-Tensae, 'AIDS, Security, and the Military in Africa: A Sober Appraisal', *African Affairs*, 105(419) (2006): 201–18; and Tony Barnett and Gwyn Prins, 'HIV/AIDS and Security Fact, Fiction & Evidence', A Report to UNAIDS (London School of Economics AIDS, for UNAIDS, 2005). The idea that rising HIV predicts conflict is in B. Bennett et al., 'HIV Incidence Prior To, During, and After Violent Conflict in 36 Sub-Saharan African Nations, 1990–2012: An Ecological Study', *PLoS ONE* 10(11) (November 2015).

The thinking on natural disasters comes from N. Veenstra, A. Whiteside, D. Lalloo, and A. Gibbs, 'Unplanned Antiretroviral Treatment Interruptions in Southern Africa: How Should We Be Managing These?', *Globalization and Health* 6(4), doi:10.1186/1744-8603-6-4. (2010).

The data from the Afrobarometer are available from <www.afrobarometer.org>.

The original analysis in Alan Whiteside, Robert Mattes, Samantha Willan, and Ryann Manning, 'Examining the HIV/AIDS Epidemic in Southern Africa through the Eyes of Ordinary Southern Africans', Afrobarometer (2003), Working Paper No. 21.

The thoughts on sovereignty are from A. Šehović, *HIV/AIDS and the South African State: Sovereignty and the Responsibility to Respond* (Ashgate, 2014).

Chapter 7: Treatment and prevention dilemmas

The idea of waves of public health is from S.C. Davies et al., 'For Debate: A New Wave in Public Health Improvement', *Lancet* 384 (April 2014).

The UNAIDS publications are the UNAIDS-Lancet Commission, 'The UNAIDS-Lancet Commission on 'Defeating AIDS–Advancing Global Health', *Lancet* (June 2015): 5.

UNAIDS, 'How AIDS Changed Everything. MDG 6: 15 Years, 15 Lessons of Hope from the AIDS Response', UNAIDS, retrieved from <http://www.unaids.org/sites/default/files/media_asset/ MDG6Report_en.pdf>.

UNAIDS, 'Thailand Ending AIDS: Thailand's AIDS Response Progress Report', retrieved from <http://www.unaids.org/sites/ default/files/country/documents/THA_narrative_report_2015.pdf>.

UNAIDS, 'On the Fast-Track to End AIDS by 2030: Focus on Location and Population', UNAIDS (2015). Retrieved from <http:// www.unaids.org/en/resources/documents/2015/ FocusLocationPopulation>.

I am grateful to Mead Over for his thinking on AIDS transitions that I have adapted. The most accessible version of this is: <http://www. cgdev.org/publication/achieving-aids-transition-preventing-infections-sustain-treatment-cgd-brief>.

WHO, 'HIV Prevention Based on ARV Drugs' (June 2013) retrieved from <http://www.who.int/hiv/pub/guidelines/arv2013/clinical/ prevention/en/index3.html>; and more recently, 'WHO Guideline on When to Start Antiretroviral Therapy and on Pre-exposure Prophylaxis for HIV', World Health Organization (2015).

The Norman Fowler book, *AIDS: Don't Die of Prejudice* (London: Backbite Publishing, 2014) was referred to as a basic introduction text.

The hotspot mapping is documented in A. Vandormael et al., 'Use of Antiretroviral Therapy in Households and Risk of HIV Acquisition in Rural KwaZulu-Natal, South Africa, 2004–12: A Prospective Cohort Study', *Lancet Global Health*, DOI: http://dx.doi.org/10.1016/S2214-109X(14)70018-; F. Tanser et al., 'Localized Spatial Clustering of HIV Infections in a Widely Disseminated Rural South African Epidemic', *International Journal of Epidemiology* (March 2009), DOI:10.1093/ije/dyp148; S. Otage, 'Uganda: How Health Units Curbed HIV Spread from Mother to Child', *All Africa* (August 2015), retrieved from <http://allafrica.com/stories/201508171131.html>.

International Partnership for Microbicides, retrieved from <http://www.ipmglobal.org/>; STRIVE, retrieved from <http://strive.lshtm.ac.uk/about>; D.B. Garone et al., 'High Rate of Virological Re-suppression among Patients Failing Second-line Antiretroviral Therapy Following Enhanced Adherence Support: A Model of Care in Khayelitsha, South Africa', *Southern African Journal of HIV Medicine* 14(4) (December 2013): 170–6; E. Chingoni, 'Malawi: Art Clients Urged to Go for Viral Load Test to Examine Drug Effectiveness', *All Africa*, retrieved from <http://allafrica.com/stories/201508180885.html>.

V. Nobel and J. Parle, '"The Hospital Was Just Like a Home": Self, Service and the "McCord Hospital Family"', *Medical History* (April 2014), retrieved from <http://www.ncbi.nlm.nih.gov/pmc/articles/PMC4006143/>; International AIDS Society, 'The Vancouver Consensus', International AIDS Society, retrieved from <http://vancouverconsensus.org/>; A. Whiteside, J. Cohen, and M. Strauss, 'Reconciling the Science and Policy Divide: The Reality of Scaling up Antiretroviral Therapy in South Africa', *South African Journal of HIV Medicine* (July 2015); and L. Garrett, 'Ebola's Lessons: How the WHO Mishandled the Crisis', *Foreign Affairs* (August 2015): 14–49, retrieved from <https://www.foreignaffairs.com/articles/west-africa/2015-08-18/ebolas-lessons>.

Chapter 8: Funding the epidemic

The data in this chapter are drawn from the following sources: United Nations Economic and Social Council, 'Joint and Co-Sponsored United Nations Programme on Human Immunodeficiency Virus/Acquired Immunodeficiency Syndrome', ECOSOC (1994), retrieved from <http://www.un.org/documents/ecosoc/res/1994/eres1994-24. htm>; UNAIDS, 'How AIDS Changed Everything. MDG 6: 15 Years, 15 Lessons of Hope from the AIDS Response', UNAIDS, p. 187, retrieved from <http://www.unaids.org/sites/default/files/ media_asset/MDG6Report_en.pdf>; S. Resch, T. Ryckman, and R. Hecht, 'Funding AIDS Programmes in the Era of Shared Responsibility: An Analysis of Domestic Spending in 12 Low-income and Middle-income Countries', *Lancet Global Health*, (2015): 52–61; Results for Development retrieved from <http:// resultsfordevelopment.org/>.

The Rethink HIV material includes P. Collier, O. Sterck, and R. Manning, 'The Moral and Fiscal Implications of Anti-Retroviral Therapies for HIV in Africa', CSAE Working Paper (February 2015).

The roundtable event co-hosted by the Harvard T.H. Chan School of Public Health to explore the fiscal challenges of HIV. This workshop was entitled, 'From a Death Sentence to a Debt Sentence: Meeting the Challenge of Long-term Liabilities of HIV Funding'; and R. Atun et al., 'Long Term Financing Needs for HIV Control in Sub-Saharan Africa in 2015–2050: Modelling Study', *British Medical Journal* (2015).

There is a great deal written on innovative financing. A useful start is Management Sciences for Health, 'Leadership, Management, and Sustainability Program 2005–2010 Final Report', USAID & MSH (2014), retrieved from <http://projects.msh.org/projects/lms/Results/ upload/LMS-final-report-12-13-10_web.pdf>.

Chapter 9: Big issues and major challenges

UNAIDS's 2015 report is remarkable in that it is realistic and focused; much of the data in the conclusion is drawn from this, 'On the Fast-Track to End AIDS by 2030: Focus on Location and Population', UNAIDS (2015), retrieved from <http://www.unaids.org/en/ resources/documents/2015/FocusLocationPopulat>.

Index

Index

THE HISTORY OF MEDICINE
A Very Short Introduction
William Bynum

Against the backdrop of unprecedented concern for the future of health care, this Very Short Introduction surveys the history of medicine from classical times to the present. Focussing on the key turning points in the history of Western medicine, such as the advent of hospitals and the rise of experimental medicine, Bill Bynum offers insights into medicine's past, while at the same time engaging with contemporary issues, discoveries, and controversies.

www.oup.com/vsi

SEXUALITY
A Very Short Introduction
Veronique Mottier

What shapes our sexuality? Is it a product of our genes, or of
society, culture, and politics? How have concepts of sexuality
and sexual norms changed over time? How have feminist
theories, religion, and HIV/AIDS affected our attitudes to sex?
Focusing on the social, political, and psychological aspects of
sexuality, this *Very Short Introduction* examines these
questions and many more, exploring what shapes our sexuality,
and how our attitudes to sex have in turn shaped the wider world.
Revealing how our assumptions about what is 'normal' in
sexuality have, in reality, varied widely across time and place,
this book tackles the major topics and controversies that still
confront us when issues of sex and sexuality are discussed:
from sex education, HIV/AIDS, and eugenics, to religious
doctrine, gay rights, and feminism.

www.oup.com/vsi

INFECTIOUS DISEASES
A Very Short Introduction
Marta L. Wayne and Benjamin Bolker

As doctors and biologists have learned, to their dismay, infectious disease is a moving target: new diseases emerge every year, old diseases evolve into new forms, and ecological and socioeconomic upheavals change the transmission pathways by which disease spread. By taking an approach focused on the general evolutionary and ecological dynamics of disease, this *Very Short Introduction* provides a general conceptual framework for thinking about disease. Through a series of case studies, Benjamin Bolker and Marta L. Wayne introduce the major ideas of infectious disease in a clear and thoughtful way, emphasising the general principles of infection, the management of outbreaks, and the evolutionary and ecological approaches that are now central to much research about infectious disease.

www.oup.com/vsi

SOCIAL MEDIA
Very Short Introduction

Join our community
www.oup.com/vsi

- Join us online at the official Very Short Introductions
  Facebook page.
- Access the thoughts and musings of our authors with our
  online **blog**.
- Sign up for our monthly **e-newsletter** to receive information
  on all new titles publishing that month.
- Browse the full range of Very Short Introductions online.
- Read **extracts** from the Introductions for free.
- If you are a teacher or lecturer you can order inspection
  copies quickly and simply via our website.

EPIDEMIOLOGY
A Very Short Introduction
Rodolfo Saracci

Epidemiology has had an impact on many areas of medicine;
and lung cancer, to the origin and spread of new epidemics.
and lung cancer, to the origin and spread of new epidemics.
However, it is often poorly understood, largely due to
misrepresentations in the media. In this *Very Short Introduction*
Rodolfo Saracci dispels some of the myths surrounding the
study of epidemiology. He provides a general explanation of
the principles behind clinical trials, and explains the nature of
basic statistics concerning disease. He also looks at the ethical
and political issues related to obtaining and using information
concerning patients, and trials involving placebos.